T0323823

'Klein and Yzerbyt's book is a valuable window on the societal dimensions of vaccination which surround individual vaccine decisions. Emotions, rumours, risk, trust and altruism are among the mix of influences that this very important book examines in the context of vaccination'.

Heidi J. Larson, *Professor of Anthropology, Risk and Decision Science; Director, The Vaccine Confidence Project, London School of Hygiene & Tropical Medicine; and Visiting Professor, Centre for Evaluation of Vaccines, University of Antwerp, and KU Leuven Belgium*

THE PSYCHOLOGY OF VACCINATION

Why do some people choose to be vaccinated and others do not? What is the difference between vaccine hesitancy and anti-vaccinism? What can social psychology tell us about attitudes towards vaccination?

The Psychology of Vaccination identifies the social psychological drivers of vaccine mindsets, to explore why some people choose to be vaccinated, some are hesitant, and others refuse. It explores the socio-demographic factors related to vaccine hesitancy and considers the role of motivation in making this health decision. The book focuses on how individuals are social beings, inserted into a web of influences that guide their behaviour, and considers the impact this may have on their health choices.

Not only aimed at the convinced, but also for all those who have doubts about vaccination, The Psychology of Vaccination offers an insightful look at our health behaviours and considers whether it is possible to affect health behaviour change.

Olivier Klein is a professor of social psychology at the Université libre de Bruxelles, Belgium.

Vincent Yzerbyt is a professor of social psychology at the Université catholique de Louvain, Belgium.

They were both involved in the "motivation barometer", a large-scale project that tracked attitudes towards vaccination (and other health behaviours) across the COVID-19 pandemic in Belgium.

THE PSYCHOLOGY OF EVERYTHING

People are fascinated by psychology, and what makes humans tick. Why do we think and behave the way we do? We've all met armchair psychologists claiming to have the answers, and people that ask if psychologists can tell what they're thinking. *The Psychology of Everything* is a series of books which debunk the popular myths and pseudo-science surrounding some of life's biggest questions.

The series explores the hidden psychological factors that drive us, from our subconscious desires and aversions, to our natural social instincts. Absorbing, informative, and always intriguing, each book is written by an expert in the field, examining how research-based knowledge compares with popular wisdom, and showing how psychology can truly enrich our understanding of modern life.

Applying a psychological lens to an array of topics and contemporary concerns – from sex, to fashion, to conspiracy theories – *The Psychology of Everything* will make you look at everything in a new way.

Titles in the series:

The Psychology of Democracy
by Darren G. Lilleker and Billur Aslan Ozgul

The Psychology of Counselling
by Marie Percival

The Psychology of Travel
by Andrew Stevenson

The Psychology of Attachment
by Robbie Duschinsky, Pehr Granqvist and Tommie Forslund

The Psychology of Running
by Noel Brick and Stuart Holliday

The Psychology of the Teenage Brain
by John Coleman

The Psychology of Time
by Richard Gross

The Psychology of Vaccination
by Olivier Klein and Vincent Yzerbyt

For more information about this series, please visit: www.routledge textbooks.com/textbooks/thepsychologyofeverything/

THE PSYCHOLOGY OF VACCINATION

OLIVIER KLEIN AND VINCENT YZERBYT

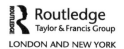

LONDON AND NEW YORK

Cover Image: © Getty Images

First published 2024
by Routledge
4 Park Square, Milton Park, Abingdon, Oxon OX14 4RN

and by Routledge
605 Third Avenue, New York, NY 10158

Routledge is an imprint of the Taylor & Francis Group, an informa business

British Library Cataloguing-in-Publication Data
A catalogue record for this book is available from the British Library

ISBN: 978-1-032-66541-2 (hbk)
ISBN: 978-1-032-66540-5 (pbk)
ISBN: 978-1-032-66542-9 (ebk)

DOI: 10.4324/9781032665429

Typeset in Joanna
by Apex CoVantage, LLC

CONTENTS

INTRODUCTION TO VACCINE HESITANCY

Sebastian is a school teacher. In his view, the COVID-19 epidemic is an invention to implement world population control (the "Great Reset"). In his view, this would be done through vaccines equipped with microchips and, if people refuse to be vaccinated, through a "COVID *passport*". Sebastian does not trust the "mainstream" media. They are controlled by the financial elites, whose vast project feeds on the fears of the population. Sebastian therefore prefers to consult alternative media, on YouTube and Facebook. It goes without saying that he didn't get vaccinated. He is too attached to his freedom to accept being put on file in this way.

Idriss, 20 years old, is unemployed. His parents have long been applying for public housing. He lives with his parents and two younger brothers and a sister in a small flat. The lockdown was particularly difficult in such a tight space. Family members have been subjected to numerous checks by the police. In these conditions, Idriss is not happy about the injunctions to be vaccinated: he faces little risk from COVID-19. Why make an effort for a society that pays so little attention to his fate? Furthermore, he does not trust the medical system. Every time a member of his family goes to hospital, it costs much more than expected and the bills pile up.

DOI: 10.4324/9781032665429-1

Amy, 32, is a midwife. She has always cultivated a lifestyle that is as environmentally friendly as possible. In particular, she only consumes organic products from a short supply chain and favours a vegetarian diet. She is convinced that the best way to stay healthy is to live as close to nature as possible, not only through a balanced diet, but also by using the resources found in plants and by exercising. This, she says, strengthens her natural immunity, as does the practice of meditation. Under these conditions, she sees no point in a vaccine, as this product of the pharmaceutical industry only confers artificial immunity.

Gabriela, 42, is a single mother of three children. She has a full-time job as a worker in a canning factory located an hour away from her home by public transport. Her mother is seriously ill and neither her father, who died two years ago, nor her two sisters, who live abroad, can help with the care. Gabriela is not opposed to vaccination, but she is so busy with her activities that she did not take the time to respond to the letter about her vaccine appointment and finds it difficult to reconcile the trip to the vaccination centre outside the city with her schedule.

Simon, 51, is an executive in a private company. Having read many texts written by experts (or people claiming to be experts) on social networks and blogs, he considers mass vaccination to be a bad idea, which only benefits pharmaceutical companies. It should be reserved for those truly at risk. The rest of the population should be left to get infected in order to develop herd immunity.

Alia, 28 years old, is a domestic helper. She is originally from Sudan. She has not been vaccinated against COVID-19 even though a vaccine has been available for her age group for over a year. According to her, by being "pricked", she will be injected with the disease. However, she considers that if she contracts COVID-19, it is Allah's will and her decisions must be accepted.

Octavia, 27, a computer scientist, is convinced of the importance of vaccination and encourages her family to get vaccinated. She, however, does not take the plunge because she has been scared to death of syringes since she was a child. As soon as she sees a nurse approaching her with the dreaded object, her blood runs cold and she almost faints. She knows it's irrational, but she can't help it.

You may recognize these fictional profiles (although inspired by real people). We imagine each of them evolving in very different worlds. Some, like Sebastian and Amy, are resolutely opposed to vaccination, out of conviction. Others, like Idriss and Gabriela, are not fundamentally against it, but want to show their distrust of the authorities (like Idriss) or simply have other priorities (like Gabriela). As we can see, the reluctance to be vaccinated can respond to very different motivations.

In 2019, vaccine hesitancy was described by the World Health Organisation (WHO) as one of the top ten threats to global health (alongside Ebola, climate change and antimicrobial resistance . . .).[1] The WHO used the term "vaccine hesitancy" to describe the refusal or reluctance to be vaccinated despite the availability of a vaccine. Experts from this respected institution attributed the resurgence of infectious diseases such as measles to such reluctance, at least in part. Since 2019, the COVID-19 pandemic has only accentuated the importance of this phenomenon, exposing significant resistance to vaccination.

Yet, in terms of public health, immunisation is one of the greatest achievements of the 20th century (WHO, 2013). For example, the WHO estimated in 2013 that childhood immunisation saved between 2 and 3 million people each year (WHO, 2013). An assessment in late 2021 estimated that COVID-19 vaccines saved nearly 750 000 lives in Europe and the United States alone.[2] Another study, published in the summer of 2022[3] and conducted in more than 185 countries around the world (with the notable exception of China), estimated that COVID-19 vaccination could have prevented 19.8 million of a potential 31.4 million deaths in the first year after the introduction of the vaccines on 8 December 2021. Yet, according to the WHO, there is significant opposition to vaccination in many parts of the world. For some diseases, immunisation rates, which had been growing rapidly up to that point, have stagnated or even fallen, partly because of resistance to the medical technology. Given its success, it seems paradoxical that there is such resistance.

The benefits of vaccination, whether at the individual or collective level, depend on the behaviour of individuals, and therefore on psychology. The issue of vaccine hesitancy has been the subject of sustained attention by researchers in psychology and what is now known as the "behavioural sciences". Work on this topic is leading to the hope of identifying possible solutions to this huge public health challenge.

Unsurprisingly, this behaviour is part of a complex system involving various institutions (national and even supranational government authorities, supervisory authorities, etc.) and funding sources (governement, insurance companies, employers, etc.) as well as a multitude of individuals (general practitioners, nurses, etc.). Each of these stakeholders, whether organisations or individuals, may have different objectives.

In this book, we approach vaccine hesitancy through the prism of social psychology. What does this mean? How does this discipline position itself in the vast landscape of the social sciences and humanities, at the crossroads of psychology and sociology? Of course, we examine the psychological factors that lead the individual to engage (or not) in a vaccination process. But far from looking at the individual in isolation, we consider him or her as a social being, inserted into a web of influences and affiliations that guide his or her behaviour, even if the behaviour is ultimately individual.

This book seeks to identify the psychosocial drivers of vaccine attitudes. Even if, as you will have understood, we believe that vaccination is a major advance in terms of public health, we hope to have succeeded in depicting the more "hesitant" postures, whether they are related to inertia, uncertainty or frank opposition, in the most objective and respectful way possible. This book is therefore not only for the convinced, but also for all those who have doubts about vaccination in general or about specific vaccines.

In this respect, it is important to emphasise the distinction between anti-vaccine attitudes and vaccine hesitancy. The former is to be understood first and foremost as an attitude likely to lead to a refusal to be vaccinated. If, according to the WHO definition, such an attitude does contribute to vaccine hesitancy, it is by no means the only possible cause. Thus, vaccine hesitancy is not necessarily based on a structured discourse against vaccination. Sometimes, as the above examples illustrate, vaccine hesitancy is based on nothing more than a lack of desire to get vaccinated or difficulty in finding the time to go to the vaccination centre. Moreover, in many cases, anti-vaccine attitudes are directed at a wide range of vaccines, if not all. Hesitancy can be much more selective, affecting, for example, certain vaccines at certain times for some patients. For example, during the COVID-19 pandemic, one of the most commonly used justifications for opposing newly developed vaccines was that "we lack hindsight". By this they meant that they were willing to accept other, well tested vaccines.

In keeping with our approach, we will treat anti-vaccinism primarily as a psychological reality – an individual or collective posture towards vaccination – but will not propose an in-depth analysis of anti-vaccination social movements, which would require a sociological analysis. As this is beyond the scope of this book and the competence of its authors, we have refrained from venturing into this field.

Vaccination offers protection against viruses and bacteria by mimicking an infection in order to stimulate natural immunity. Their effectiveness often relies on booster doses, as individual immunity can decline over time. Some vaccines, such as those for influenza, require an annual dose because the pathogens change from year to year. In addition to the individual protection that vaccines provide, they also reduce the circulation of pathogens within a community. Herd immunity is achieved when enough members of a group are vaccinated so that the pathogen can no longer reproduce.

The term "vaccination coverage" refers to the proportion of people vaccinated against a disease in a population at a given time. The vaccine coverage required to achieve herd immunity depends on the disease and its degree of contagiousness. For example, for measles, a potentially deadly disease, 95% coverage is required. In the US, this percentage hovers around 90% and is much lower in some communities. It is hardly surprising that a measles outbreak occurred in 2019.

From a psychological point of view, it is important to emphasise that vaccination coverage – the fact of being effectively vaccinated for a sufficiently large proportion of the population – requires the implementation of active behaviour on the part of individuals. This behaviour must be *motivated*. The motivation to be vaccinated precedes the behaviour. Of course, the nature of this behaviour may vary in complexity and in the effort required. In some cases, vaccination requires only signing a document authorising the child to be vaccinated at school. In other cases, getting vaccinated means making an initial appointment with a doctor and then going to a vaccination centre or hospital far from home. In this respect, a distinction can be made between *accepting* a proposed vaccine and *actively seeking* one. While the former is more common in countries of the global North where major vaccines are routinely offered, the latter is more common in less affluent countries, where many vaccines are not immediately offered and require a much more active approach to secure their administration.

Where does the term "vaccine hesitancy" fit in this context? The term is widely used in the literature to refer to the lack of willingness to be vaccinated. However, the term can refer to:

- an attitude: when we speak of "reticence" or even "mistrust";
- Motivation: hesitation may reflect a lack of motivation to be vaccinated, and in some cases a motivation not to be vaccinated;
- a behaviour: when talking about "refusal".

The term "vaccine hesitancy" is therefore used to refer to quite different psychological realities. This does not help to organise the already dense literature on the subject. In this volume, we will consider vaccine hesitancy as essentially a *motivational issue*. A continuum can be drawn from a strong motivation not to vaccinate (or not to vaccinate one's child) to a strong motivation to vaccinate (or to vaccinate one's child). Vaccine hesitancy is therefore the counterpart of the motivation to be vaccinated. Motivation then leads to actual behaviour (getting vaccinated or having the child vaccinated).

After an initial overview of the socio-demographic factors related to vaccine hesitancy, we will look more closely at the psychological mechanics of vaccination, focusing on the individual. We will then broaden the focus to the social and collective dimension in Chapters 3 and 4. Before concluding, Chapter 5 will examine a series of avenues for reducing vaccine hesitancy.

NOTES

1 www.who.int/news-room/spotlight/ten-threats-to-global-health-in-2019.

2 Mallapaty, S., Callaway, E., Kozlov, M., Ledford, H., Pickrell, J., & Van Noorden, R. (2021). How COVID vaccines shaped 2021 in eight powerful charts. *Nature*, 600(7890), 580–583.

3 Watson, O. J., Barnsley, G., Toor, J., Hogan, A. B., Winskill, P., & Ghani, A. C. (2022). Global impact of the first year of COVID-19 vaccination: A mathematical modelling study. *The Lancet Infectious Diseases*, 22(9), 1293–1302.

1

WHO ARE THE VACCINE HESITANT?

When asked who the "vaccine hesitant" or "anti-vaxxers" are, one often hears two types of answers. One refers to psychological characteristics: are these people more or less intelligent than others? More paranoid? More anxious? The other type refers to sociological or demographic factors: are these people more or less educated? More economically vulnerable? Do they work in certain professions? Are they mostly found in specific age categories? In this chapter we will try to identify vaccine hesitancy from a socio-demographic point of view.

However, a word of caution is in order before embarking on this task. As we shall see, indicators of vaccine hesitancy, and even statistics on actual vaccine uptake, can obviously be linked to information on the characteristics of those who hesitate. Indeed, it is not uncommon to observe links between socio-demographic variables and these indicators. However, when interpreting these relationships, it is important to bear in mind that they are statistical relationships and in no way justify 'stereotyping' some categories of people as uniformly "anti-vaxx". For example, if there is a negative relationship between education level and vaccine hesitancy, this does not mean that people with low levels of education or even that a majority of

DOI: 10.4324/9781032665429-2

them refuse vaccination. The data simply show that there are proportionally fewer people opposed to vaccination as education level increases. It may even be the case that at all levels of education, vaccination is the majority option. Moreover, as we shall see, these relationships are likely to vary depending on the vaccine being considered[1] and the context. With these caveats in mind, let us try to identify some "strong trends" in the relationship between demographic factors and vaccine hesitancy.

SOCIAL CLASS

Historically, opposition to vaccination has been particularly prevalent among the working classes.[2] Numerous surveys confirm a greater prevalence of this stance among people of relatively low socioeconomic status.[3]

One explanation is that the less educated (education being one of the criteria defining "social class") are more likely to "fall through the cracks" of vaccination campaigns. This is sometimes due to logistical difficulties. To take a factor that may seem trivial: the invitation must arrive at the right address! The most disadvantaged people are more likely to live in temporary housing or not to have reported their address to the local authorities. There may also be a difficulty in understanding written instructions due to low literacy levels.

As we will see in the following chapters, a range of psychological factors may also come into play: the first is less trust in institutions and authorities. The least educated people are also statistically likely to feel the least close to the authorities and the least well represented by them. This can fuel a form of mistrust and cast doubt on their good intentions in implementing a vaccination campaign.

Another aspect concerns the perception of greater vulnerability. Indeed, when people are deprived of material resources, they often feel more at the mercy of possible external dangers. A vaccine, despite its possible benefits, is often seen as likely to cause undesirable effects. Such fears may explain greater resistance to vaccination.

In addition, for people in precarious situations, other considerations often take precedence over the hypothetical negative consequences that the shot would prevent. Getting vaccinated requires considering the long-term effects of a disease on oneself or on the population. However, numerous studies suggest that the most disadvantaged people tend not to project themselves into the future as easily as more affluent individuals.[4] They are often busy dealing with pressing needs, which makes it difficult to consider long term plans. Such a frame of mind can prevent people from taking action on vaccination. In this case, as Gabriela's example mentioned in the introduction illustrates, it is not necessarily a matter of genuine distrust in vaccination. Simply, without being explicitly rejected, getting vaccinated appears to be less of a priority and the subsequent consequences of this decision are hardly considered with as much attention.

Despite this body of evidence, it should be emphasised that it is not always people from working-class backgrounds who are most likely to shy away from a vaccine. This depends in particular on the vaccine under consideration. For example, in a study conducted in 2010[5] in France, although the least educated people were generally the most reluctant to be vaccinated, it was individuals with an intermediate level of education (bachelor's degree) who were the most opposed to the H1N1 vaccine. For COVID-19, another French survey[6] found greater opposition to the vaccine among those with no degree or a general secondary degree than among those with a vocational degree (with those with higher degrees being even less resistant).

The effect of social class on vaccine hesitancy may also vary depending on whether one is deciding on one's own vaccination or that of one's children. In the latter case, people are likely to be particularly attentive to the potential long-term risks of choosing to vaccinate (or not). Studies suggest that educated parents are sometimes the most likely to refuse vaccination for their offspring.[7] In addition to the greater propensity to consider long-term outcomes that is characteristic of the affluent, this may also be explained by a distrust of science and its potential abuses. Vaccines are the result of complex technologies that very few people master. The fact that they involve the injection of viral components can make them particularly worrying. Some parents (often from the "middle class") are therefore especially fearful of the dangers posed by such technological advances.

Note that when we talk about social class, we often think of two indicators: income level and education level. In this case, these two factors do not have the same impact on vaccine hesitancy. It seems that it is mainly the level of education that plays a role in vaccination – even if there is also reluctance to vaccinate in privileged circles. This is not surprising because, as we shall see, attitudes towards vaccination depend very much on the socialisation process. Schooling obviously plays an important role.

RELIGION

The relationship between religiosity and vaccine hesitancy is another theme worthy of interest. Historically, the fight against vaccination has often been led by religious organisations, which saw the disease as a divine destiny.[7] In 2019, measles cases exploded in some parts of New York City due to the refusal of members of the Orthodox Jewish community to be vaccinated. The belief that health is a divine prerogative sometimes justifies some of these positions. But while people may oppose vaccination on religious grounds, the links between religiosity and vaccine hesitancy are weak or absent. For example, a study of parents of 2-year-olds in the United States (mostly from very low-income and migrant backgrounds) found no link between membership in any of the major monotheistic religions and vaccine hesitancy.[8] Religiosity, i.e. investment in faith (which may be manifested, for example, by attending religious services), was also unrelated to hesitancy.

In this respect, beyond the convictions and practices of each individual, it is important to take into account the mobilizing power of the *leaders* of religious institutions. The link between the sacred texts on which a faith is based and the issue of vaccination is often far from obvious. This is not surprising, since vaccination emerged long after the texts. It is therefore a matter of interpretation and it goes without saying that the views of religious authorities play a large role in the decision of the faithful to be vaccinated or not.[9] However, it is remarkable that individuals' decisions sometimes run counter to those of religious authorities. For example, in an American study,[10] ultra-Orthodox Jewish mothers who consulted their rabbi on a wide range of everyday decisions did not do so, or even defied the rabbi's recommendations, when it came to vaccinating their children. Indeed, most rabbis in this community were in favour of vaccinating children.

GENDER

Does the reluctance to vaccinate affect women and men equally? Historically, vaccination was closely linked to patriarchy. Vaccination campaigners were usually men who sought to vaccinate children, whose care was the prerogative of women. In a context where the world of medicine and medical practices (dominated by men and "controlling" women's bodies) seemed overtly sexist, it is not surprising that the fight against vaccination was seen as a feminist struggle by some feminist leaders. Today, despite changing gender relations, women still play a greater role in caring for children, who are primarily concerned by vaccination. As a result, the weight of mothers is greater than that of fathers in the decision in this matter.[11] In France for example, there is a (slightly) greater opposition to vaccination among women. In fact, this tendency is particularly noticeable in relation to COVID-19.[12]

Several explanations have been put forward to account for this (very small) difference. On average, women would be more socialised to appreciate a "natural" lifestyle, "close to the body". Such a conception is perceived as antithetical to vaccination, which is seen as a technological intrusion into the "natural" functioning of the body. Women are also more concerned about the potential dangers of vaccination in relation to pregnancy and their children. More generally, the relationship to health has changed over time. Medical users are less and less passive. Patients are no longer content to listen passively to what a professional tells them and apply it scrupulously. From the end of the 20th century a much more active vision has developed. Each person becomes an active agent who informs himself/herself autonomously and seeks from health professionals a dialogue informed by his/her own research. People want to be involved in all medical decisions. These more active patients are often women. They play a major role in household health decisions, especially those concerning children.

AGE

Surveys on attitudes towards vaccination always include a question on age. Is there a relationship between age and vaccine hesitancy? This hypothesis is particularly relevant for people of legal age, who are required to make an individual decision about vaccination.

In general, older people are more supportive of vaccination. This relationship can be partly explained by their greater vulnerability. However, the trend is not necessarily linear. In a French study,[13] younger women (25–34 years) were the most hostile to vaccination and acceptance of vaccination increased after 45 years. This may be because they were more concerned about adverse effects of vaccination during pregnancy.

ETHNICITY AND CULTURAL BACKGROUND

Studies in Western European countries tend to find greater resistance to vaccination among people of African, and particularly sub-Saharan, immigrant background. In the United States, too, there is significant resistance in African-American communities. There are many reasons for this resistance, but one of the most common factors cited is that these communities are (or feel) often marginalised from the health care system. Historically, they have been victims of ethically reprehensible practices that may have left a mark on collective memory. One example is the syphilis experiments conducted in

Tuskegee, Alabama, between 1932 and 1972, which used exclusively African-American populations as human guinea pigs. Other experiments were conducted by Western companies (including Pfizer) in sub-Saharan Africa without respecting ethical prescriptions (such as informed consent) that would have been impossible to avoid in the North.

In France, opposition to vaccination is also more pronounced among people from the overseas territories or those of African or Asian origin. During the COVID-19 pandemic, the vaccination rate remained particularly low in Guadeloupe and Martinique. In November 2021, there were even protests and a general strike following the mandatory vaccination of health workers. The distance from institutions in mainland France and the resulting mistrust could explain such attitudes, which are also fuelled by disinformation spread on social networks.

Obviously, since people from immigrant backgrounds and certain ethnic minorities are often represented in the working classes, it is particularly difficult to dissociate the role of the level of education from the cultural factor in explaining vaccine hesitancy among these groups. And this is without taking into account the religious factor, which may also play a role.

CONCLUSION

At the end of this rapid inventory based on a few classic socio-demographic indicators, it is clear that the profile is rather vague and will be of limited use to investigators seeking to explain insufficient vaccination coverage. Certainly, low socio-economic status, belonging to an ethnic or cultural minority and youth seem to be factors associated with vaccine hesitancy, but the links observed in the various studies on the subject are often tenuous and variable. Indeed, if there is one constant trend in the literature on vaccine hesitancy, it is inconsistency. The trends are shifting and change or even reverse depending on the context, the vaccine under consideration, the country, etc. And make no mistake about it, there is vaccine hesitancy in all social environments. It is not a disposition firmly anchored in the personality of individuals and determined once and for all by their membership in a sociological group. As we shall see, beyond the strictly psychological factors, vaccine hesitancy is part of a social psychological dynamic and must be interpreted rather as an individual's positioning in relation to a given situation in a given social context.

NOTES

1 Smith, M. J., & Marshall, G. S. (2010). Navigating parental vaccine hesitancy. *Pediatric Annals*, 39(8), 476–482.

2 Durbach, N. (2000) 'They might as well brand us': Working-class resistance to compulsory vaccination in Victorian England. *Social History of Medicine*, 13(1), 45–63.

3 Peretti-Watel, P., Raude, J., Sagaon-Teyssier, L., Constant, A., Verger, P., & Beck, F. (2014). Attitudes toward vaccination and the H1N1 vaccine: Poor peoples unfounded fears or legitimate concerns of the elite? *Social Science & Medicine*, 109, 10–18.

4 Mullainathan, S., & Shafir, E. (2013). *Scarcity: The true cost of not having enough.* New York: Holt.

5 Peretti-Watel, P. et al. (2014). *Op. cit.*

6 Bajos, N., Spire, A., Silberzan, L., & Group for the E study. (2022). The social specificities of hostility toward vaccination against Covid-19 in France. *PLOS One*, 17(1).

7 Salvadori, F., & Vignaud, L.-H. (2019). *Antivax: la resistance à la Vaccination du XVI-IIème ciècle à nos jours* [Antivax: Resistance to vaccines from the 18th century to the present dayI]. Paris: Vendémiaire.

8 Williams, J. T. B., Rice, J. D., & O'Leary, S. T. (2021). Associations between religion, religiosity, and parental vaccine hesitancy. *Vaccine: X*, 9, 100121.

9 Dubé, È., Ward, J. K., Verger, P., & MacDonald, N. E. (2021). Vaccine hesitancy, acceptance, and anti-vaccination: Trends and future prospects for public health. *Public Health*, 42, 175–191.

10 Keshet, Y., & Popper-Giveon, A. (2021). "I took the trouble to make inquiries, so I refuse to accept your instructions": Religious authority and vaccine hesitancy among ultra-orthodox Jewish mothers in Israel. *Journal of Religion and Health*, 60(3), 1992–2006.

11 Wu, A. C., Wisler-Sher, D. J., Griswold, K., Colson, E., Shapiro, E. D., Holmboe, E. S., & Benin, A. L. (2008). Postpartum mothers' attitudes, knowledge, and trust regarding vaccination. *Maternal and Child Health Journal*, 12(6), 766–773.

12 Bajos, N. *et al.* (2022). *Op. cit.*

13 *Ibid.*

2

PSYCHOLOGICAL DETERMINANTS OF VACCINATION IN INDIVIDUALS

Given the scale of the COVID-19 pandemic, a logical, simple and effective measure was to vaccinate the entire population. At the same time, it has always seemed unimaginable that government authorities would opt for a generalised vaccine mandate. The pitfalls of such an approach are not limited to issues of monitoring the proper application of the measure and the possible sanction in the event of non-compliance, far from it. Since the use of variolisation, vaccinia[1] and then the vaccine itself, resistance has always been many and varied. A fortiori, in the cultural and ideological environment of Western societies at the beginning of the 21st century, the population intends to be offered the possibility of being vaccinated on the basis of a free choice. In this context, vaccination is bound to be based on a range of psychological factors, the most important of which is individual motivation.

Unsurprisingly, the motivational dimension of behaviour is at the heart of a very rich array of models in psychology. For many authors,[2] while many factors can affect the decision to vaccinate, motivation is the most direct – proximal – determinant of vaccine intention and its negative counterpart, vaccine hesitancy. In addition to motivation, other variables play a role in shaping vaccine hesitancy. These factors,

DOI: 10.4324/9781032665429-3

referred to as "distal", have an impact on vaccine hesitancy via their influence on motivation. This chapter focuses on the more individual, psychological determinants.

PROXIMAL FACTORS: INTENTION AND MOTIVATION

Intention − that is, the decision to vaccinate − is a prerequisite for vaccination. For adults or parents of children of vaccination age, intention is a necessary condition for vaccination. Much research in health psychology therefore studies the determinants of vaccine intention in the hope of understanding vaccination itself. However, the relationship between intention and behaviour is not mechanical. Think of people who have firmly decided to lose the kilos they gained during the winter and look desperately at their weighing scale a few months later. An intention is all the more informative if it relates to a specific and temporally proximate context: "i intend to get vaccinated at 8:30 a.m. on Saturday at the Franklin Avenue vaccination centre" is a better indicator of actual behaviour than "I intend to get vaccinated once the safety of the vaccines is established". In short, the word "intention" can have multiple psychological meanings! In the remainder of this chapter, we will refer to an intention to be vaccinated in the short term.

Intention is determined by *motivation*, which is the impetus that gives purpose or direction to the behaviour. In order to form the intention to be vaccinated, one must first be *motivated* to be vaccinated. One of the most celebrated approaches to motivation in social psychology, self-determination theory (SDT), was developed by Deci and Ryan.[3] The sense of autonomy, the feeling of being in control of one's actions, of enjoying full independence in the choices one makes in the face of life's circumstances plays a central role. Other psychological scientists had already highlighted the crucial role played by the conviction that one is not just the plaything of events but can, on the contrary, act as one pleases. Thus, according to reactance theory,[4] any attempt to restrict a person's freedom of action will provoke a response whose primary objective will be to restore one's sense of autonomy and, *ultimately*, one's freedom of action. This psychological principle is used extensively in our daily lives, especially in advertising and marketing: stating that a film is forbidden to under-18-year-olds is a sure way to arouse the curiosity of teenagers.

In the perspective of SDT, autonomy is viewed as a basic psychological need whose satisfaction serves the development and well-being of the person.[5] Individuals engage in a behaviour because they are convinced of its necessity and of its associated benefits. In this context, people identify with vaccination and subscribe to the idea that it increases protection of self and others. Autonomous motivation indicates that individuals have internalized the reasons for vaccination. Indeed, along with three other basic needs – competence, relatedness and security – the satisfaction of the autonomy need accounts for a substantial part of the sense of well-being of citizens during this pandemic.[6]

An international survey[7] of over 5,000 people in 24 countries illustrates the major role of this need for autonomy. The authors examined the psychological determinants of attitudes towards vaccination. They included measures of autonomy in their questionnaire. For example, how much their respondents agreed with statements such as "I find contradicting others stimulating "or "I consider advice from others an intrusion". This variable was found to be strongly related to vaccination attitudes: a high level of agreement was associated with a very negative attitude towards vaccination. These results illustrate the desire to preserve one's freedom in the face of vaccination campaigns perceived as restrictive and the role it can play in vaccine hesitancy. This analysis will come as no surprise to observers of anti-vaxx movements, the health *pass* and/or compulsory vaccination that emerged during the COVID-19 pandemic: freedom was their mantra.

From a SDT perspective, these basic needs are not so much culturally specific as they are universal. Numerous studies attest to the central role of this feeling of autonomy and the motivation that accompanies it, particularly in the case of smoking,[8] diabetes[9] or eating habits.[10] Table 2.1 provides an overview of the basic needs and subjective experiences associated with their satisfaction and frustration.

Table 2.1 Basic needs

Need	**Satisfaction**	**Frustration**
Autonomy	Sense of volition and psychological freedom	Sense of pressure and psychological conflict
Relationship	Sense of connection and attention	Sense of exclusion and isolation
Competence	Sense of effectiveness and control	Sense of failure and inadequacy
Security	Sense of predictability and certainty	Sense of uncertainty and powerlessness

Conversely, the challenge to this autonomy is accompanied by the experience of constraint and frustration. This is called *controlled* motivation. People act but feel pressure to perform the behaviour to escape criticism and disapproval. They may also bend to the promised rewards if they comply. According to SDT, such a situation obviously generates a range of costs. These include feelings of unhappiness, psychological difficulties and even reactance. Indeed, some people may feel that they are required to silence their doubts about the efficacy of the vaccine and get vaccinated without a second thought in order to fulfil their civic duty. This context may contribute to the emergence of mistrust of the invitation to vaccinate.

Just as motivation for vaccination is multifaceted, lack of motivation may be due to a range of reasons. There are two types of "amotivation", one rooted in distrust and the other in effort. The first type is rooted in distrust and the second in effort. The distrust-related amotivation reflects the doubts that individuals have about the vaccine. These doubts concern first and foremost the safety and efficacy of the vaccine itself. In fact, the action of the vaccine and its possible side effects are essential drivers of vaccine hesitancy.[11] Furthermore, the presumed intentions and competence of the health professionals and authorities promoting vaccination also fuel the distrust of the public.[12]

Effort fatigue refers to the fact that some people do not have all the resources, either psychological or physical, to carry out their desire to be vaccinated.[13] For example, people may feel lost when trying to make

Table 2.2 Types of motivation and amotivation for vaccination

Why do you want to be vaccinated?			
De-motivation	Controlled motivation, "Mustivation"		Autonomous motivation, "want-ivation"
Discouragement, Caution	Expectations, punishment, rewards	Shame, guilt, self-questioning.	Personal values
I don't want to devote the effort	Otherwise I will be sanctioned	Otherwise, I will Feel guilty	It makes sense
I don't think that the current approach is working	Otherwise, I will be criticized	It is the only way to be satisfied with myself	I understand the merits of vaccination

an appointment to be vaccinated. They may also not have access to transport to special vaccination sites or be unable to attend vaccination centre opening hours. Table 2.2 provides an overview of the different types of motivations related to vaccination. An ideal situation would be to have all the people on the right side of the table. Actually, many people are more likely to be found in the left-hand boxes. Despite this, and the SDT-inspired research makes this abundantly clear, a significant number of less motivated or even recalcitrant individuals move to the right as the evolution of the situation allows for ownership of the desired behaviours and understanding of the reasons supporting them. There is then an increase in the sense of autonomy through internalisation and empowerment. Unsurprisingly, some people will remain reluctant lacking autonomous motivation.

While the role of voluntary and controlled motivations is well established for a wide range of health behaviours, research on vaccine uptake using the theoretical framework of SDT is still in its infancy. Some work has shown that frustrating respondents' autonomy is indeed related to vaccine refusal.[14] Recent studies carried out in Belgium in the context of the Motivation Barometer[15] allow for a better appreciation of the role of different types of motivation and amotivation on the intention to be vaccinated as well as on the uptake of the vaccine a few months later.

Box 2.1   The Motivation Barometer

The Motivation Barometer (http://motivationbarometer.com) is an inter-university project initiated by Ghent University (Belgium) from the beginning of 2020 and bringing together scholars from different subfields of psychology (social psychology, health psychology, motivational psychology, etc.). It was soon joined by colleagues from the Katholieke Universiteit Leuven, the Université catholique de Louvain and the Université libre de Bruxelles. This tool made it possible to monitor fluctuations in motivation and other social psychological variables in the Belgian population throughout the pandemic. In some two years and forty successive waves of data collection, no less than 400,000 responses were collected. The numerous reports resulting from this barometer made it possible to inform the population and the media as well as the authorities and other expert groups about the psychological issues related to the COVID-19 crisis. The studies carried out within this framework have also led to numerous scientific publications.

For example, in a cross-sectional study conducted between November and December 2020, just as the vaccination campaign was about to be launched, Schmitz and colleagues[16] examined the vaccination intentions of almost 9,000 unvaccinated Belgian citizens. One of the central concerns of the study was the link between motivation and vaccination intention. The questions focused on autonomous motivation, controlled motivation, effort motivation and distrust motivation. For example, autonomous motivation was measured by questions such as "Getting vaccinated is in line with my personal values", "I fully agree with getting vaccinated", "It makes a lot of sense for me to get vaccinated". The ambition was to assess the extent to which each type of motivation "predicts" vaccination intention. Autonomous motivation was found to be by far the most important predictor. This was followed by motivation rooted in lack of trust, which affected vaccine intention, but this time in a negative way. Controlled motivation and effort-related amotivation also play a role, but to a much lesser extent, although the relationship remains significant.

A second study, this time longitudinal, made it possible to refine these results. After an initial measurement period between 20 December 2020 and 31 January 2021, a second survey was carried out between 21 and 31 May 2021, gathering the complete data of nearly 7, 000 respondents who were divided into two samples, depending on whether the persons had already received an invitation (some 5, 800 responses) or not (nearly 1, 200 responses). In the first case, it is possible to investigate the role of the motivations at time 1 on the actual taking of the vaccine at time 2. In the second case, we can examine the impact of the motivations at time 1 on registration on a waiting list in order to benefit from a vaccine as soon as possible. It should be noted that at this stage of the vaccination campaign, the sending of an invitation was mainly based on the age and co-morbidity conditions of the persons concerned. As in study 1, the results are clear. They highlight the massive role of autonomous motivation measured at time 1 on the fact of being vaccinated or of having registered on the waiting lists at time 2. While controlled motivation seems to have a very modest impact on actual vaccination among those who received an invitation, the other types of motivation have no significant impact on behaviour.

These data are impressive, to say the least, as they highlight the crucial role of autonomous motivation in vaccine intention. A clear message from these studies is that vaccination is not rooted in controlled types of motivation involving internal or external pressures.

Box 2.2   Does the effectiveness of a vaccine depend on psychological factors?

In this book we focus on the social psychological aspects of vaccine hesitancy. This might suggest, wrongly, that once people agree to be vaccinated, these aspects play little role. An

American study[17] shows that this would be a serious mistake. In this study, university students were administered a flu vaccine (corresponding to three different antigens). They were then followed for four months. The authors were particularly interested in two important variables: the size of their social network (the number of people with whom they were in regular contact) and their feelings of loneliness. Note that these two variables cover different realities: one can feel lonely even if one meets many people and *vice versa*. It turns out that these two variables predicted the effectiveness of the vaccine: the antibodies linked to one of the antigens were indeed produced in smaller quantities in the most isolated people and in those who felt the loneliest. The data from this study suggest that stress, caused in part by loneliness, may inhibit antibody production. Although the mechanisms responsible for these results are still mysterious, they show that the effectiveness of vaccination, even once the barrier of hesitation has been overcome, is still influenced by psychological factors.

DISTAL FACTORS: TRUST

One of the most common approaches to vaccine hesitancy in the literature is the "3Cs" approach.[18] This typology lists the factors that shape the degree of hesitancy of people in their vaccination process. The abbreviation refers to the roles of *confidence*, *complacency* and *comfort* as key factors. We examine these aspects in turn.

Trust is undoubtedly the aspect that has most engaged the attention of researchers, policymakers and the general public. People are more likely to be vaccinated if they believe that the vaccine is sufficiently effective and safe.[19] The information we have, receive and seek about the advantages and disadvantages of vaccination is the basic material that shapes our attitudes towards vaccines. To speak of attitudes is basically to speak of confidence, which can be defined as follows:

> A relationship between individuals, as well as between individuals and a system, in which one party accepts a vulnerable position, assuming the best interests and competence of the other, in exchange for a reduction in decision complexity.[20]

To trust is to accept to put one's fate in the hands of others – in this case, those who develop, recommend and administer a vaccine.

CONFIDENCE IN THE EFFICACY AND SAFETY OF THE VACCINE

Vaccination is anything but trivial. It involves being injected a product that most of us know nothing about. We do not have the expertise to know exactly what the vaccine is made of and how it was produced. This is especially important in the case of some COVID-19 vaccines, as they appear to use a revolutionary technology (such as messenger RNA). Let's face it, we also know and understand less and less about what is in most everyday consumer products, be they ready-made meals, cleaning and hygiene products, or of course medicines. The renewed interest in sustainable, local and organic consumption reflects this perplexity, which can sometimes be observed, albeit in an exacerbated form, in relation to vaccines.

In order to be accepted, a vaccine must be perceived as safe and effective. Together, these two aspects drive the level of public confidence. Confidence is expressed as a positive attitude rooted in beliefs about the various features of the vaccine, and these attitudes then shape the intention to be vaccinated. Work in social psychology confirms that attitudes towards a vaccine are the most relevant antecedents of intentions to vaccinate.[21] These demonstrations support the findings of a myriad of studies conducted within social-cognitive models of health behaviour such as the theory of reasoned action[22] and the theory of planned behaviour (TPB).[23]

The idea common to these two approaches is simple: a behaviour, such as vaccination, is the result of a behavioural intention, in this case the intention to be vaccinated. This intention is itself rooted both in a more personal ground (an attitude), and in a more social soil, a subjective norm. The attitude summarises the knowledge of the various consequences, some positive and others negative, attached to the performance of the behaviour but also the probability of their occurrence. For example, we imagine that getting vaccinated entails a significant risk of a feeling of pain at the site of the injection. In the end, this pitfall is not very negative, even if it is highly certain. One can also consider the hardly disputable fact that one will have to travel to a vaccination centre (or to the doctor). This may not be a problem for some, but it may be a much greater cost for others. Consideration of these elements, namely the advantages and disadvantages of the behaviour and their likelihood, will shape the intention to engage in this behaviour.

The subjective norm refers to the beliefs that individuals hold about the positions attributed to various sources of influence with respect to behaviour and the extent to which one intends to conform or not to these sources. For example, Mr. Campbell may believe that his life partner does not support vaccination and may feel it prudent to conform to this view. In this case, the intention to be vaccinated may be weakened. On the other hand, he or she will learn how much good his or her family doctor thinks about vaccination. If they are generally keen to adopt their family doctor's recommendations, then these will have a positive impact on their intention to be vaccinated. But there may be other factors involved. For example, the country's authorities may advocate vaccination through well publicized campaigns, leaving no doubt as to their position on the matter. However, if Mr. Campbell gives only moderate credit to the political world, this will have the effect of tempering the implementation of the behaviour.

The most recent of the two theories considered here, the TPB, proves to be highly relevant in the present context, as it highlights the joint role of attitudes and social norms, but also adds that of perceived control, all of which have a high degree of overlap with the notions of confidence, complacency and comfort, respectively, of the 3C model. Let's take a closer look at attitudes, which are a serious candidate for predicting vaccination intentions.

In a study of the human papillomavirus vaccine (HPV),[24] Caso and colleagues[25] measured Italian parents' intentions *not* to use the HPV vaccine, but also their attitudes towards non-vaccination, their perceived control, and anticipated regret, i.e. the degree to which respondents expected to regret their decision in the event of non-vaccination (we will return to this concept of anticipated regret later). In addition, the researchers probed negative attitudes towards the vaccine, risk perception, but also trust in institutions and science, and what these authors called "religious morality". The data confirm the primary role of attitudes about vaccination as a predictor of intention not to vaccinate. These attitudes are themselves strongly rooted in negative attitudes towards the vaccine.

In view of this pattern, the question remains whether this status of attitudes as a prelude to intentions also manifested itself in the context of the COVID-19 pandemic. This question was precisely addressed in a study conducted in April 2021 among a large sample of Germans.[26] Once again, attitudes proved to be the main determinant of vaccination intentions. Interestingly, the results already mentioned in Chapter 1 emerge with regard to demographic variables. Indeed, being older, male rather than female, indigenous, and having a higher level of education leads to more positive attitudes. But, related to the point at hand, these are also rooted in vaccine scepticism. The more people say they are sceptical about the vaccine, the less positive their attitudes and the less they report an intention to be vaccinated. These results therefore fully support the picture described above.

D(M)ISINFORMATION AND TRUST

In the spring of 2020, both the WHO Director General and the UN Secretary General stated that the "fight" against our "common enemy" is not only about the COVID-19 pandemic but also about the "infodemic" of misinformation.[27] The concept of infodemic refers to the presence of too much information, some of which is genuine and some of which is false. Such a flow, which the Internet makes possible, would be difficult for consumers to manage and would lead them to implement behaviours harmful to public health. The term "infodemic" is used by analogy with that of an epidemic, as if the spread of false information were equivalent to that of a virus. This analogy is misleading. Viruses spread from one individual to another and often unintentionally. In contrast, the dissemination of false or misleading information about immunisation is driven by communities and even institutions with identifiable objectives. Viewing the spread of misinformation as a disembodied epidemic obscures this fundamental reality.

Every citizen is confronted with information about vaccination. This information can come from health authorities but also from acquaintances, various influencers or activist groups. They can be communicated by word of mouth, through the mainstream media or through social networks. Some are scientifically backed up, others completely unfounded. And there is a spectrum between these two extremes. Before discussing the consequences of this abundance of information, it is important to define some concepts and in particular the distinction between "misinformation" and "disinformation".[28] Disinformation is deliberately misleading information. In contrast, misinformation refers to information that is false but not intended to deceive.

Some people or institutions knowingly communicate incorrect information about vaccines, or do not care about their accuracy. This is the case of websites seeking to create as much "click bait" as possible in order to increase the rate of engagement and their advertising revenues or who wish to market various alternatives to treatments recognised by the scientific community. It is also done by some political actors using disinformation to mobilise audiences in line with their interests. For example, the Russian[29] government had been found to finance real companies producing disinformation ("troll farms"), in particular via "*bots*", i.e. automated programmes posing as real users and flooding social networks with messages. One study looked at the content of vaccine-related communications issued by bots.[30] It appears that while these bots send out "anti-vaxx" content, they also relay a "pro-vaccination" discourse. The aim of those who program this software is not so much to provoke mistrust of vaccination as to encourage polarisation and conflict.

There are two main categories of misinformation about vaccination.[31] The first is the claim that vaccines are responsible for various diseases (autism, multiple sclerosis, etc.) and that they cause adverse effects. This type of discourse is fuelled by a view of science as being untrustworthy because of disagreements between scientists and the evolution of knowledge. Both elements create uncertainty and give credence to a discourse that emphasises the risks of the vaccine.

A second category concerns conspiracy theories suggesting that pharmaceutical companies and health authorities are covering up the reality about vaccine (lack of) effectiveness and (lack of) security. This is a misunderstanding of the scientific process, according to which knowledge is only established if 100% of scientists agree with it. It also equates undisputed knowledge (the overall efficacy of vaccines) with debates on current and unresolved scientific issues.

Other forms of disinformation concern the effectiveness of vaccines, which are said to be less useful than expected and/or that alternatives (e.g. via nutrition or homeopathic treatments), would be much more effective. Disinformation can also dispute the seriousness of diseases. Who has not heard that COVID-19 was just a "little flu"? For some infectious diseases that vaccination has succeeded in curbing, we are faced with a paradox: it is because the said disease has virtually disappeared *thanks to vaccination* that it no longer gives rise to much fear, or even seems benign. Indeed, in most cases, measles and mumps cause only mild symptoms, but the rare serious or even fatal cases justify high vaccination coverage.

Other actors communicate inaccurate information in good faith, convinced that their advice on vaccination is sound. This is known as "misinformation". As knowledge about vaccination evolves, what is "information" at one point may later become "misinformation" or "disinformation".

Studies on misinformation show that knowledge of, or exposure to, such misinformation is related to vaccine hesitancy.[32] In other words, people who see a lot of these "fake news" on their screens are less enthusiastic about vaccination than those who see little. However, this does not prove a causal relationship. As we will see below, merely having an attitude about an issue makes us more likely to seek out information consistent with that attitude.[33]

Social psychology research suggests that misinformation is difficult to resist.[34] For example, in a study conducted at the University of Brussels,[35] subjects were asked to listen to an account of a crime. This was provided by a woman and a man who, each, reported parts of the account. The subjects were explicitly told that the information given by one of the two speakers (e.g., the woman) was false. Following this account, the subjects were asked to suggest a judicial sentence for the defendant. The authors varied the nature of the false information: for half of the subjects, it was a mitigating circumstance, for the other half, an aggravating circumstance. The authors found that participants in the "aggravating" condition proposed harsher sentences than those in the "mitigating" condition, even though they knew the information was false. In addition, they were administered a memory test consisting of identifying whether the information they had been presented with previously was true or false. Their memory was of course not perfect. But it was oriented: subjects were much more likely to misidentify false information as true than to consider true information as false. Thus, information influences our judgements even when we know it is false and that when we are exposed to false information, we tend to forget that it is false.

This truth bias is explained by a tendency in our minds to treat all information as true *a priori*. We often think of ourselves as sceptics who follow Cartesian doubt. In this view, we do not believe information if there is no reason to believe it. In fact, this study suggests that we tend to adhere to information as soon as we are exposed to it. Philosophy buffs will have recognised a reality more akin to what Spinoza proposes to us. It is only in a second stage, and with some effort, that we are able to reject information as false. Such an effort requires motivation and cognitive resources. Who has the desire or the energy to check the veracity of every piece of information to which he or she is exposed?

The evidence is clear: the impact of misinformation on vaccination attitudes is cause for concern. Unlike the subjects of this study, people who are confronted with false information about vaccination are not warned and their vigilance is therefore likely to be minimal. A large study[36] (over 8,000 subjects) conducted in the US and the UK in 2020 (before the start of vaccination campaigns) examined attitudes towards COVID-19 vaccination before and after subjects were exposed to five pieces of misinformation about risks of adverse effects from vaccination (e.g. the idea that vaccines change RNA, or that they are designed to decrease the size of the world's population). Another group was exposed to five factual and truthful pieces of information about the vaccines then in preparation (control group). While there was no change in vaccination intentions in the control group, the decrease in the percentage of people who were definitely willing to be vaccinated was about 6% in the group exposed to misinformation. This percentage was observed just after exposure to misinformation and, although of concern, it suggests that this brief exposure had a relatively limited short-term effect. However, in the context of such a study, respondents are probably more focused and alert than they would be in more natural situations.

Based on the work on the truth bias, the effect of this misinformation is explained by the difficulties our cognitive system encounters to be "vigilant". The beliefs that would be instilled as a result of misinformation would come to influence our attitudes and behaviours towards vaccination. In particular, misinformation about vaccines leads to an increased perception of risk,[37] which is hardly surprising when it calls into question their safety.

However, misinformation does not only influence our beliefs, but also our emotions. This is particularly important in the case of vaccination: to be vaccinated is to accept that a stranger injects you with a substance (at the cost of pain and possible side effects) to prevent a potentially dangerous disease. All of these aspects are emotionally charged. Vaccine misinformation often seeks to mobilise emotions by showcasing victims of adverse vaccine reactions, especially children and infants. Who would be confident after seeing a little girl paralysed or suffering from an incurable disease after taking a vaccine?

Which emotions are we talking about? Fear is certainly the most important. Fear of adverse effects can undermine any motivation to get vaccinated. Another emotion is anger. This emotion may stem from the frustration of being told to vaccinate (especially if it seems unjustified) and the feeling of being duped by the authorities. In a study conducted in 2020,[38] US subjects were presented with various messages about vaccination. In the first condition (uncertainty), inducing the first category of misinformation mentioned above, the (ostensible) uncertainties of the scientific community on this issue were highlighted. In a second condition (conspiracy), inducing the second category, information was presented about a conspiracy between governments and pharmaceutical companies to hide the influence of the MMR vaccine[39] on autism. In a control condition, a message unrelated to vaccination was presented. Unsurprisingly, participants exposed to both misinformation conditions expressed less positive attitudes towards the vaccine. Why? In the conspiracy condition, subjects reported more fear than in the control condition. However, this increase in fear did not explain the effect of this form of misinformation on attitudes towards the vaccine. In contrast, in both conditions (conspiracy and uncertainty), there was an increase in anger, which in turn accounted for the difference in attitudes towards MMR vaccination compared to the control condition. Thus, it appears that anger is a more effective vector of de-motivation with respect to vaccination than fear.

TRUST AND ITS SOURCES

Mass vaccination is a massive undertaking that involves a chain involving multiple agents: the political authorities who decide to implement it, the scientists who develop knowledge about infectious diseases necessary for the development of vaccines, the universities in which they work, the researchers who develop the vaccines, often within pharmaceutical companies, the companies that manufacture them, the institutions that control the safety of the vaccines, the distribution networks that make sure that they are kept in good conditions and are not altered, right down to the people (nurses, doctors . . .) who inject the product. Imagine that only one of these actors has bad intentions or seems unable to execute his task: it is very likely that you would then hesitate to run the risk of being injected with a potentially dangerous product. It is impossible to be sure that all agents in this vast system are honest, caring and competent. To agree to be vaccinated, you must either have sufficient contempt for yourself and your health, or you must find it rational and acceptable to assume that these actors are sufficiently competent and benevolent to inject you with an effective and safe product. The credit you give to the actors in this system is, of course, trust.

Rumours, conspiracy theories and anti-vaccine social representations have the effect of undermining this confidence. In 1998, Bernard Kouchner, then Minister of Health in the French government, suspended the systematic vaccination against hepatitis B in schools because of suspected cases of multiple sclerosis due to it. In doing so, he was at odds with WHO experts who emphasised the extreme rarity of these cases compared to the benefits of the vaccine. A link between this vaccine and hepatitis B was be established, but the long-term effect on vaccination coverage were disastrous.

Suppose that trust in one of the agents in the chain that enables mass vaccination is lost. This may call into question other agents. Consider a vaccine being produced under poor conditions by an unscrupulous company. If this vaccine is nevertheless marketed, it will call into question confidence in the authorities that have encouraged its distribution and the supervisory bodies that have validated it. The fact that vaccination also involves financial transactions can, of course, contribute to mistrust. When this is the case, recovery becomes extremely difficult.

In this respect, the episode of the H1N1 vaccination campaign in France in 2009 is particularly telling. In the early 2000s, opinion polls showed widespread support for vaccination among French people (over 90%). Following the H1N1 epidemic, the Minister of Health, Roselyne Bachelot, ordered tens of millions of doses of the vaccine from pharmaceutical companies. The campaign was an abject failure, partly because the epidemic turned out to be much less severe than expected. This fiasco raised suspicions of conflict of interest and fuelled conspiracy theories: why spend so much money on a vaccine that is useless? The Mediator scandal[40] also contributed to this belief in collusion between the authorities and pharmaceutical laboratories. The result: in 2010, 40% of French people considered themselves to be rather unfavourable to vaccination (this rate was 8.6% in 2000[41]). This rate of mistrust has subsequently remained very high, making France one of the countries in Europe where vaccine hesitancy is the highest.

The attitude towards vaccination often reflects a more general attitude towards the authorities. It can be a roundabout way of expressing disapproval of policies that have little to do with health. In 2019, a Pakistani government official called for a boycott of polio immunisation until electricity was regularly installed in his region.[42] Vaccination is often seen as a dictate from distant authorities whose concerns are far removed from the more pressing concerns of those they are targeting. Refusing to vaccinate is tantamount to expressing spite and even resentment towards such contemptuous authorities.

In the case of COVID-19, surveys conducted across the world confirm that trust in the authorities and health system actors is one of the main determinants of vaccination.[43] For example, in a study conducted in Belgium in early 2021,[44] trust in the authorities was an important predictor of intention to vaccinate. People who trusted the authorities showed a higher *autonomous* motivation to get vaccinated. In other words, they saw this choice as a deliberate decision on their part: it made sense, whether from the point of view of their own health, that of their loved ones or of public health as a whole.

The greater self-motivation of those who trusted the authorities explained their willingness to be vaccinated. When one has faith in the authorities, one is willing to put oneself in the hands of health professionals and accept vaccination as a deliberate choice, not as an external imposition. Trust in the authorities did not indeed translate into greater controlled motivation, and the latter had only a very weak effect on vaccination intentions.

Beyond government authorities, what about trust in other actors? Most people are rarely in frequent contact with their government authorities or academic experts on vaccination. Instead, people are more likely to visit their general practitioner, to be in contact with nurses in hospitals or at home, or to go to the pharmacy. Given their proximity, these health system actors are likely to enjoy greater trust. For example, people who are reluctant to be vaccinated often listen to their general practitioner. When parents who are reluctant to have their child vaccinated change their mind, it is generally because their GP's advice has paid off.[45] In fact, the main source of information on vaccines is usually the doctor, far ahead of the Internet.[46]

However, not everyone trusts the health sector. There is a fear that doctors are themselves biased or influenced by concerns other than patients' health. In a study conducted in the Netherlands,[47] one element that differentiated parents who were reluctant to vaccinate from those who were not was their confidence in the information provided by their doctor: they were more likely to feel that their doctor was only extolling the benefits of vaccination and was unaware of its drawbacks. Health professionals must therefore be objective and sensitive to parents' fears about the potential risks of vaccination. Sometimes, distrust in one's doctor is less about bias than about incompetence. For example, a young Brussels resident interviewed by Maes[48] said that he did not trust a doctor practising in a neighbourhood medical practice because consultations were free: "the doctor who works there is not good, otherwise he would be a specialist and he would earn a lot of money".[49]

While doctors play an important role in supporting vaccination, it is important not to underestimate the number of doctors who express significant reservations about vaccination as a whole or about some commonly administered vaccines. For example, in a study conducted on a large sample of French general practitioners,[50] there was overwhelming support for vaccination but a sizeable proportion of respondents (between 16% and 43% depending on the vaccine considered) admitted that they did not recommend vaccines on a regular basis to their patients. This lack of support was explained by a lack of trust in the government and medical institutions responsible for vaccination. In short, general practitioners did not behave differently from the rest of the population.

Confidence in medicine as a discipline also plays an important role in adherence to vaccination. After all, vaccination is a product of "traditional" medicine, as taught in universities. A study[51] examined this idea by asking a representative sample of the Spanish population about their attitudes towards vaccination as well as their views on conventional medical practices (chemotherapy and antidepressants). The authors found a strong link between vaccine hesitancy and distrust of these practices. This was true not only for users of "conventional" medicine, but also for those who preferred "natural" medicines (homeopathy, acupuncture, etc.). Behind the hesitation to vaccinate may therefore lurk a more general mistrust of conventional medicine.[52]

In sum, our analysis of the role of trust in vaccination allows us to resolve a paradox: how is it that attitudes towards vaccination are generally positive when "fake news" about the supposed risks of vaccines abound? Shouldn't the truth bias make people susceptible to such claims and therefore deeply suspicious? The resolution of this conundrum lies in the trust that people place in certain sources: by preferentially exposing themselves to trusted sources, individuals can drastically limit their exposure to a variety of information, whose level of credibility may vary. Trust appears to be a remarkable tool of cognitive economy: it prevents us from having to deal with a mass of information that is of no interest or that comes from dubious sources. It turns out that, when it comes to immunisation, the sources that are most trusted by the public are those that are most reliable. We have talked about health workers, but if we turn to the media, we see that the "traditional" media also enjoy the highest level of trust.[53] As a result, the deleterious effects of the truth bias are reduced. Pockets of vaccine hesitancy will be found among individuals or groups who do not trust the mainstream media and/or conventional medical actors. In such an informational microcosm, "fake news" will be much more numerous. It will therefore be more difficult to detect them as such[54] and, even if they are, the truth bias is likely to promote much more anti-vaccine attitudes.

DISTAL FACTORS: COMPLACENCY

In the 3C model, complacency refers to the way people approach the situation, and in this case to a form of inertia towards the vaccination decision. This passivity occurs when the risks associated with the disease are perceived to be low and the vaccine is therefore not seen as necessary to avoid them.[55]

RISK PERCEPTION

The issue of risk assessment is central to vaccination. Numerous studies show that risk perception plays a major role, both in terms of the perceived probability of infection, i.e. the risk of being infected, and the perceived severity of infection, i.e. the severity of the infection. A review of the literature on influenza vaccine hesitancy shows that the perception of a low risk[56] of contracting influenza is the most important barrier to influenza vaccination in almost 10% of the 470 studies considered.

The Motivation Barometer studies unambiguously establish risk perception as a major lever in the adoption of protective measures. For example, Schmitz and colleagues[57] asked respondents about their subjective estimation of the likelihood of being infected with COVID-19 and of becoming seriously ill as a result of such an infection. These risk perceptions, measured in January 2021, were positively related to vaccination or to being placed on a waiting list, measured in May 2021. These effects were fully explained by the influence of risk perception on autonomous motivation. In other words, when someone perceives the risks to be important, they feel more intrinsically motivated to get vaccinated, which then predicts actual vaccination. Interestingly, this study also sheds some light on the distinction between risk perception and related concepts such as worry about COVID-19. Risk perception refers to an estimate of probability and not to an emotional state, like worry. In this study, worry related to COVID-19, measured by items such as "During the past week, during the Covid crisis, I have been worried about my health", did not predict vaccination when risk perception was also taken into account. Thus, it is subjective risk perception, not anxiety or fear, that drives motivation to get vaccinated.

In fact, throughout the COVID-19 pandemic, citizens showed a high sensitivity to more or less alarmist information from official sources, especially regarding hospitalisation and intensive care unit stays. A study,[58] again in the framework of the Motivation Barometer, supports this idea. We recorded the level of perceived risk (in terms of likelihood and severity of a COVID-19 infection) continuously for twenty months (from June 2020 to March 2022). The average perceived risk level (in terms of severity) in the sample followed the hospitalization statistics. In turn, levels of autonomous motivation to adopt health measures and vaccination were predicted by this risk perception, confirming the data of Schmitz and colleagues. Such a result argues for a "rational" approach to communication about vaccination: rather than scaring people, it is important to provide them with clear guidance about the risks of infection.

In this respect, two important elements should be noted. One constant in the communication of the authorities during this pandemic has been to talk about variations in the reproduction rate (R) and the increase (or decrease) in infections, hospitalisations, intensive care bed occupancy and even deaths over time. All of this may help to motivate the population to support the health measures advocated by authorities. However, a major handicap in assessing the evolution of risks lies in the fact that the human brain has a very poor grasp of both the exponential nature of the evolution of contamination and the baseline levels.

UNDERSTANDING EXPONENTIAL FUNCTIONS

A salient feature of a pandemic is the importance of an accurate assessment of the progression of the disease in the population. People have very little difficulty in understanding arithmetic progressions, i.e. progressions in which the same number is always added to the previous number. This is also known as linear growth. Things get very bad with exponential progressions. In these cases, it is no longer the addition that is constant but the ratio between a number and the previous number. In a study conducted at the start of the COVID-19 pandemic (in January and February 2020) on a representative sample of the US population,[59] the fictitious scenario was presented of an illness where one person was infected on the first day, transmitted the virus to two other people the next day before stopping being contagious . . . and so on. So it was an exponential transmission. The subjects were asked to estimate how many people would be infected on days 5, 10 and 20. How would you answer? Take a moment to think about this. Most people might think that a threefold increase in the number of cases per day is not dramatic. Indeed, the median responses[60] from participants were 16, 30 and 60, indicating that people thought the epidemic was growing in a linear fashion. And while some realised that it was probably more and increased their estimate accordingly, a tiny minority of respondents were able to guess the correct answer, namely 31, 1,023 and over a million, respectively!

As we can see, the reproduction rate, R, appears deceptively reassuring. When it is around 1.81 (one person infects an average of 1.81 others), to take an example that sometimes occurred during the pandemic, this still yields a sizeable group of more than 4,000 people infected after a fortnight, and this from a single case. In many ways, this difficulty in identifying the disastrous effects of a single infection may have contributed to minimising the willingess to vaccinate. In the case of COVID-19, preventive measures (e.g., social distancing) and vaccinaton could greatly reduce the spread of the virus.

BASE RATES AND NARRATIVE BIAS

You see a young woman reading poems by Lord Tennyson on a bench next to the market near your home. Incongruous question: is she a historian specialising in medieval history or a cleaning lady (you have to choose between these two options)? To answer this question, one is tempted to rely solely on the stereotype (reading old poems is more in keeping with the profile of a person with an intellectual profession). This ignores an important factor, the so-called 'base rates': there are many more female cleaning ladies than specialists in medieval history. If there are 10, 000 cleaning ladies in your city and 100 medieval historians, you are *a priori* 100 times more likely to see a cleaning lady in a public square than a historian – literary preferences should have a small weight in your answer compared to this statistical 'sledgehammer'. And yet, when base rates are available, people tend to overlook them when they also have information that is consistent with or contrary to stereotypes about particular individuals.[61] It is as if the individual reality overshadows the general trends.

The same phenomenon applies to hospitalization figures when one chooses to report the number of cases among vaccinated and unvaccinated persons. Indeed, as a vaccine never offers 100% protection, some vaccinated persons are included in the hospitalization cohort. These few cases of vaccinated people getting sick anyway can completely overshadow the effect of these statistics. We may know that, in general, the vaccine protects against disease (so the baselines tell us), but an exemplary an idiosyncratic case that goes against the norm leaves more of an impression. A good story is more influential than statistics – this is called "narrative bias", a bias that influences vaccination intentions.[62] Hence the importance of not presenting vaccines as an absolute shield, as some politicians have sometimes done at the beginning of vaccination campaigns, even though they protect well against infection and mild forms of the disease and are very effective against severe forms of COVID-19.

One element amplifies the influence of singular examples: our tendency to consider two consecutive events (e.g. getting vaccinated

islands, devoid of connection to others. Deliberately or not, members of a given population shape the behaviour of others as much as they prove sensitive to what they see around them. The next chapter looks at how social influences affect the decision to vaccinate.

NOTES

1 Variolisation is the voluntary inoculation of smallpox from a weakly ill person in order to prevent it. It is a technique that dates back to ancient China and is based on the same principle as vaccination. Vaccinia is a form of smallpox that particularly affects cows but can also affect humans. Edward Jenner's (1749–1823) observation that vaccinia protects against smallpox led him to inject it for preventive purposes. This is the origin of vaccines.

2 Brewer, N. T., Chapman, G. B., Rothman, A. J., Leask, J., & Kempe, A. (2017). Increasing vaccination: Putting psychological science into action. *Psychological Science in the Public Interest, 18*(3), 149–207.

3 Ryan, R. M., & Deci, E. L. (2017). *Self-determination theory: Basic psychological needs in motivation, development, and wellness.* New York: Guilford.

4 Brehm, J. W. (1966). *A theory of psychological reactance.* New York: Academic Press.

5 Vansteenkiste, M., Ryan, R. M., & Soenens, B. (2020). Basic psychological need theory: Advancements, critical themes, and future directions. *Motivation and Emotion, 44*(1), 1–31.

6 *Ibid.*

7 Hornsey, M. J., Harris, E. A., & Fielding, K. S. (2018). The psychological roots of anti-vaccination attitudes: A 24-nation investigation. *Health Psychology, 37*(4), 307–315.

8 Williams, G. C., McGregor, H. A., Sharp, D., Levesque, C., Kouides, R. W., Ryan, R. M., & Deci, E. L. (2006). Testing a self-determination theory intervention for motivating tobacco cessation: Supporting autonomy and competence in a clinical trial. *Health Psychology, 25*(1), 91–101.

9 Senécal, C., Nouwen, A., & White, D. (2000). Motivation and dietary self-care in adults with diabetes: Are self-efficacy and autonomous self-regulation complementary or competing constructs? *Health Psychology, 19*(5), 452–457.

10 Verstuyf, J., Vansteenkiste, M., Soetens, B., & Soenens, B. (2016). Motivational dynamics underlying eating regulation in young and adult female dieters: Relationships with healthy eating behaviours and disordered eating symptoms. *Psychology & Health, 31*(6), 711–729.

11 Lane, S., MacDonald, N. E., Marti, M., & Dumolard, L. (2018). Vaccine hesitancy around the globe: Analysis of three years of WHO/UNICEF joint reporting form data-2015–2017. *Vaccine*, 36(26), 3861–3867.

12 Brownlie, J., & Howson, A. (2005). 'Leaps of faith' and MMR: An empirical study of trust. *Sociology*, 39(2), 221–239.

13 Legault, L., Green-Demers, I., & Pelletier, L. (2006). Why do high school students lack motivation in the classroom? Toward an understanding of academic amotivation and the role of social support. *Journal of Educational Psychology*, 98(3), 567–582.

14 Šakan, D., Žuljević, D., & Rokvić, N. (2020). The role of basic psychological needs in well-being during the COVID-19 outbreak: A self-determination theory perspective. *Frontiers in Public Health*, 8.

15 Schmitz, M., Luminet, O., Klein, O., Morbée, S., Van den Bergh, O., Van Oost, P., Waterschoot, J., Yzerbyt, V., & Vansteenkiste, M. (2022). Predicting vaccine uptake during COVID-19 crisis: A motivational approach. *Vaccine*, 40(2), 288–297.

16 *Ibid.*

17 Pressman, S. D., Cohen, S., Miller, G. E., Barkin, A., Rabin, B. S., & Treanor, J. J. (2005). Loneliness, social network size, and immune response to influenza vaccination in college freshmen. *Health Psychology*, 24(3), 297–306.

18 Larson, H. J., Clarke, R. M., Jarrett, C., Eckersberger, E., Levine, Z., Schulz, W. S., & Paterson, P. (2018). Measuring trust in vaccination: A systematic review. *Human Vaccines & Immunotherapeutics*, 14(7), 1599–1609.

19 Xiao, X. (2021). Follow the heart or the mind? Examining cognitive and affective attitude on HPV vaccination intention. *Atlantic Journal of Communication*, 29(2), 93–105.

20 Larson, H. J. *et al.* (2018). *Op. cit.* p. 1599.

21 See for example Britt, R. K., & Englebert, A. M. (2018). Behavioral determinants for vaccine acceptability among rurally located college students. *Health Psychology and Behavioral Medicine*, 6(1), 262–276 or Cha, K.-S., & Kim, K. M. (2019). The factors related to mothers' intention to vaccinate against hepatitis A: Applying the theory of planned behavior. *Child Health Nursing Research*, 25(1), 1–8.

22 Fishbein, M., & Ajzen, I. (1975). *Belief, attitude, intention and behavior: An introduction to theory and research.* New York: Addison-Wesley.

23 Ajzen, I. (1991). The theory of planned behavior. *Organizational Behavior and Human Decision Processes*, 50(2), 179–211.

24 Human papillomavirus (HPV) is a sexually transmitted virus that can cause cervical cancer. A vaccine is available.

25 Caso, D., Capasso, M., Fabbricatore, R., & Conner, M. (2021). Understanding the psychosocial determinants of Italian parents' intentions not to vaccinate their children: An extended theory of planned behaviour model. *Psychology & Health*, 37(9), 1111–1131.

26 Seddig, D., Maskileyson, D., Davidov, E., Ajzen, I., & Schmidt, P. (2022). Correlates of COVID-19 vaccination intentions: Attitudes, institutional trust, fear, conspiracy beliefs, and vaccine skepticism. *Social Science & Medicine*, 302, 114981.

27 Bheekhun, Z., Lee, G., & Camporesi, S. (2021). Challenges of an 'infodemic': Separating fact from fiction in a pandemic. *International Emergency Nursing*, 57, 101029.

28 Pantazi, M., Hale, S., & Klein, O. (2022). Social and cognitive aspects of the vulnerability to political misinformation. *Political Psychology*, 42, 267–304.

29 Pomerantsev, P. (2019). *This is not propaganda: Adventures in the war against reality*. London: Faber & Faber.

30 Broniatowski, D. A., Jamison, A. M., Qi, S., AlKulaib, L., Chen, T., Benton, A., Quinn, S. C., & Dredze, M. (2018). Weaponized health communication: Twitter bots and Russian trolls amplify the vaccine debate. *American Journal of Public Health*, 108(10), 1378–1384.

31 Featherstone, J. D., & Zhang, J. (2020). Feeling angry: The effects of vaccine misinformation and refutational messages on negative emotions and vaccination attitude. *Journal of Health Communication*, 25(9), 692–702.

32 Neely, S. R., Eldredge, C., Ersing, R., & Remington, C. (2022). Exposure to misinformation: A survey analysis. *Journal of General Internal Medicine*, 37(1), 179–187.

33 Knobloch-Westerwick, S., & Meng, J. (2009). Looking the other way: Selective exposure to attitude-consistent and counterattitudinal political information. *Communication Research*, 36(3), 426–448.

34 Gilbert, D. T. (1991). How mental systems believe. *American Psychologist*, 46, 107–119.

35 Pantazi, M., Kissine, M., & Klein, O. (2018). The power of the truth bias: False information affects memory and judgment even in the absence of distraction. *Social Cognition*, 36(2), 167–198.

36 Loomba, S., de Figueiredo, A., Piatek, S. J., de Graaf, K., & Larson, H. J. (2021). Measuring the impact of COVID-19 vaccine misinformation on vaccination intent in the UK and USA. *Nature Human Behaviour*, 5(3), 337–348.

37 Raude, J. (2020). Vaccination: A French hesitation. *The Conversation*. https://theconversation.com/vaccination-une-hesitation-francaise-150773.

38 Featherstone, J. D., & Zhang, J. (2020). *Op. cit.*

39 Measles-mumps-rubella vaccines, which are usually given as a single injection to children (first dose around 12 months and second dose between 15 and 18 months).

40 Mediator is an anti-diabetic drug that was marketed between 1973–2009 despite serious side effects (heart damage that could lead to death), concealed by company executives and overlooked by the drug safety agency (according to the trial conducted in 2019).

41 Peretti-Watel, P., Verger, P., Raude, J., Constant, A., Gautier, A., Jestin, C., & Beck, F. (2013). Dramatic change in public attitudes towards vaccination during the 2009 influenza A (H1N1) pandemic in France. *Eurosurveillance*, 18(44), 20623.

42 Larson, H. J. (2020). *Stuck: How vaccine rumors start and why they don't go away.* Oxford, UK: Oxford University Press.

43 Casiday, R., Cresswell, T., Wilson, D., & Panter-Brick, C. (2006). A survey of UK parental attitudes to the MMR vaccine and trust in medical authority. *Vaccine*, 24(2), 177–184.

44 Van Oost, P., Yzerbyt, V., Schmitz, M., Vansteenkiste, M., Luminet, O., Morbée, S., Van den Bergh, O., Waterschoot, J., & Klein, O. (2022). The relation between conspiracism, government trust, and COVID-19 vaccination intentions: The key role of motivation. *Social Science & Medicine*, 301, 114926.

45 Gust, D. A., Darling, N., Kennedy, A., & Schwartz, B. (2008). Parents with doubts about vaccines: Which vaccines and reasons why. *Pediatrics*, 122(4), 718–725.

46 Ward, J. K., & Peretti-Watel, P. (2020). Understanding vaccine distrust: From perception biases to controversies. *Revue Française de Sociologie*, 61(2), 243–273.

47 Paulussen, T. G. W., Hoekstra, F., Lanting, C. I., Buijs, G. B., & Hirasing, R. A. (2006). Determinants of Dutch parents' decisions to vaccinate their child. *Vaccine*, 24(5), 644–651.

48 Maes, R. (2021). La spirale de la disaffiliation [The spiral of disaffiliation]. *La Revue Nouvelle*, 6(6), 2–5.

49 Ibid. p. 3.

50 Raude, J., Fressard, L., Gautier, A., Pulcini, C., Peretti-Watel, P., & Verger, P. (2016). Opening the "vaccine hesitancy" black box: How trust in institutions affects French GPs' vaccination practices. *Expert Review of Vaccines*, 15(7), 937–948.

51 Hornsey, M. J., Lobera, J., & Díaz-Catalán, C. (2020). Vaccine hesitancy is strongly associated with distrust of conventional medicine, and only weakly

associated with trust in alternative medicine. *Social Science & Medicine*, 255, 113019.

52 Van Oost, P., Schmitz, M., Klein, O., Brisbois, M., Luminet, O., Morbée, S., Raemdonck, E., Van den Bergh, O., Vansteenkiste, M., Waterschoot, J., & Yzerbyt, Y. (2022). *When views about alternative medicine, nature, and god come in the way of people's vaccination intentions.* Manuscript in preparation, Catholic University of Leuven.

53 Kantar. (2021). *Trust in news.* http://www2.kantar.com/l/208642/2017-10-27/6g28j#_ga=2.20041789.483771043.1656086215-503995251.1656086206.

54 Batailler, C., Brannon, S. M., Teas, P. E., & Gawronski, B. (2022). A signal detection approach to understanding the identification of fake news. *Perspectives on Psychological Science*, 17(1), 78–98.

55 MacDonald, N. E. (2015). Vaccine hesitancy: Definition, scope and determinants. *Vaccine*, 33(34), 4161–4164.

56 Schmid, P., Rauber, D., Betsch, C., Lidolt, G., & Denker, M.-L. (2017). Barriers of influenza vaccination intention and behavior – a systematic review of influenza vaccine hesitancy, 2005–2016. *PLOS One*, 12(1).

57 Schmitz, M. *et al.* (2022). *Op. cit.*

58 Waterschoot, J., Yzerbyt, V., Soenens, B., den Bergh, O.V., Morbée, S., Schmitz, M., van Oost, P., Luminet, O., Klein, O., & Vansteenkiste, M. (2022). How do vaccination intentions change over time? The role of motivational growth. *Health Psychology*, 42(2). Advance online publication.

59 Fetzer, T., Hensel, L., Hermle, J., & Roth, C. (2021). Coronavirus perceptions and economic anxiety. *The Review of Economics and Statistics*, 103(5), 968–978.

60 The "median" means that 50% of the sample provided a response below (or equal to) these estimates and 50% provided a response above (or equal to) these estimates.

61 Tversky, A., & Kahneman, D. (1974). Judgment under uncertainty: Heuristics and biases. *Science*, 185(4157), 1124–1131.

62 Betsch, C., Haase, N., Renkewitz, F., & Schmid, P. (2015). The narrative bias revisited: What drives the biasing influence of narrative information on risk perceptions? *Judgment and Decision Making*, 10(3), 241–264.

63 Johansen, M. K., & Osman, M. (2015). Coincidences: A fundamental consequence of rational cognition. *New Ideas in Psychology*, 39, 34–44.

64 Cho, H., Lee, J.-S., & Lee, S. (2013). Optimistic bias about H1N1 Flu: Testing the links between risk communication, optimistic bias, and self-protection behavior. *Health Communication*, 28(2), 146–158.

65 Sandberg, T., & Conner, M. (2008). Anticipated regret as an additional predictor in the theory of planned behaviour: A meta-analysis. *British Journal of Social Psychology*, 47(4), 589–606.

66 Brewer, N. T., DeFrank, J. T., & Gilkey, M. B. (2016). Anticipated regret and health behavior: A meta-analysis. *Health Psychology*, 35(11), 1264–1275.

67 Ritov, I., & Baron, J. (1990). Reluctance to vaccinate: Omission bias and ambiguity. *Journal of Behavioral Decision Making*, 3(4), 263–277.

68 Cox, D., Sturm, L., & Cox, A. D. (2014). Effectiveness of asking anticipated regret in increasing HPV vaccination intention in mothers. *Health Psychology*, 33(9), 1074–1083.

69 Meppelink, C. S., Smit, E. G., Fransen, M. L., & Diviani, N. (2019). 'I was right about vaccination': Confirmation bias and health literacy in online health information seeking. *Journal of Health Communication*, 24(2), 129–140.

70 Kunda, Z. (1990). The case for motivated reasoning. *Psychological Bulletin*, 108(3), 480–498.

71 Tang, L., Fujimoto, K., Amith, M. (Tuan), Cunningham, R., Costantini, R. A., York, F., Xiong, G., Boom, J. A., & Tao, C. (2021). "Down the rabbit hole" of vaccine misinformation on YouTube: Network exposure study. *Journal of Medical Internet Research*, 23(1), e23262.

72 Jenkins, K. (2014). II. Needle phobia: A psychological perspective. *British Journal of Anaesthesia*, 113(1), 4–6.

73 McLenon, J., & Rogers, M. A. M. (2019). The fear of needles: A systematic review and meta-analysis. *Journal of Advanced Nursing*, 75(1), 30–42.

74 Baxter, A. (2021). Over half of adults unvaccinated for COVID-19 fear needles – here's what's proven to help. *The Conversation*. https://theconversation.com/over-half-of-adults-unvaccinated-for-covid-19-fear-needles-heres-whats-proven-to-help-161636.

75 *Ibid*.

76 Love, A. S., & Love, R. J. (2021). Considering needle phobia among adult patients during mass COVID-19 vaccinations. *Journal of Primary Care & Community Health*, 12, 21501327211007390.

3

VACCINE HESITANCY WITHIN GROUPS

As soon as the availability of some COVID-19 vaccines was announced in Belgium, polls suggested that the minimum vaccination rate needed to stop the pandemic (then estimated at 70%) was unlikely to be reached. Simultaneously, many sources reported the frustration of a sizeable portion of the population who were eager to be vaccinated. Given the gradual arrival of doses, it was logically decided to make the vaccine available primarily to those most at risk of developing complications from the disease. This explains why the campaign opted for an age-tiered approach, taking into account co-morbidities. Fortunately, the production and delivery of the vaccine in early 2021 proved to be highly effective and has enabled the campaign to cover demand at an unprecedented rate. However, the issue raised by this debate between health or age-based priority and "volunteering-based" priority is fascinating and deviates from a strictly individualistic approach. It concerns the ability of vaccinated people to lead the way and to set an example for others. Indeed, the literature on this subject is plentiful[1]: individuals are far more sensitive to the behaviour of others than is generally thought.

DOI: 10.4324/9781032665429-4

VACCINATION AND SOCIAL NORMS

Social norms can be defined as a set of rules and prescriptions about how to think, feel and act. They provide reference scales that define a range of opinions or behaviours that are licensed or, on the contrary, sanctioned. For example, it is a well-established norm in our country that when invited to a friend's house for dinner, one should not come empty-handed. Some norms are even stricter, and others are even the focus of explicit rules, sometimes punishable by sanctions in the event of non-compliance. This is what happens to smokers who forget that you do not smoke in a restaurant. An impressive number of norms regulate our lives and are followed with varying degrees of success.

Two main types of norms can be distinguished.[2] *Descriptive* norms provide information about the behaviour of people around us, often those who are important to us and to whom we are willing to pay attention. These norms are markers that guide us in society and provide examples to follow. For example, if you feel that all cyclists are happily running red lights, this may inform your behaviour as a cyclist. *Prescriptive* norms are shared standards of what to do in a given situation. For example, a high level of social disapproval can be expected if someone has a laugh at a funeral. Prescriptive and descriptive norms can be distinct: one can know that driving at 30 mph in central London is a requirement (prescriptive norm), but feel that no one does it (descriptive norm).

SOCIAL PROOF AND THE KNOCK-ON EFFECT

Most often, norms preexist to individuals. They are learned during socialisation, hence the importance of the social context in which one evolves. The most critical situation in this respect is when an individual arrives in a new social environment. Such a change can significantly affect one's understanding of what are desirable and even acceptable behaviours or opinions. In a classic study,[3] American female students from rather conservative backgrounds were followed not only during their college education, but also for several decades after graduation. The institution attended was known for its politically liberal stance. The data show that the students' attitudes shifted increasingly to the left of the political spectrum as they progressed through college.

What others do, say and think therefore plays a key role in determining our own actions, words and thoughts: this is known as "social proof".[4] The importance of this phenomenon is illustrated by a process that is often neglected or even disparaged, namely imitation. It is rarely acknowledged, but the reason why human beings learn so quickly and so well is that they can draw on their extraordinary ability to capitalise on the observations of others. What others do or don't do and how these choices are sanctioned offers prime information. The psychologist Albert Bandura[5] has clearly shown how observing a person's behaviours, as long as they do not result in punishment, facilitates the emergence of identical behaviours among bystanders. Imitation and, more broadly, social proof are extraordinarily effective, sometimes in the literal sense. For example, the publication of suicides in the press or media is usually accompanied by an "unusual" increase in the number of suicides in the region concerned.[6]

But how and why do social norms have such an impact? The secret, so to speak, lies in the irrepressible tendency of human beings to compare themselves with others. How can we determine the acceptability of what we say, the correctness of what we feel, the adequacy of what we do, in short, how can we know what we are worth without looking to others and assessing whether we are on the same level or falling short? There are rarely clear criteria for judging the validity of what we think, feel or do, apart from the information we can gather from the behaviour of others. Advertisers have understood this well, as they constantly tell us that a given book is a bestseller, that a given car is the car of the year, or that a given colour is fashionable.

In the health domain, norms play an important role. A very informative study[7] examined the impact of norms on health-related intentions and behaviours by focusing on experimental studies, or randomised controlled trials (RCTs, see Box 3.1), which are best able to establish cause and effect relationships.

Box 3.1 What Is a Randomised Controlled Trial (RCT)?

Imagine the following situation: your best friend reports that she was convinced to have her daughter vaccinated by her paediatrician. The paediatrician showed her a video of a mother crying over the death of her child from a measles outbreak. Would you conclude that showing this video is an effective intervention? If so, you may be jumping the gun. We don't know if your friend would have vaccinated her child without this video and/or if another speech from her paediatrician would have had the same effect. Now imagine that you have access to a large number of parents, some of whom you know have seen the video and some of whom have not. You also learn that more people who saw the video got their child vaccinated than those who did not. Does this prove that the video was effective? Not necessarily. I is possible that parents who bothered to watch the video were already more supportive of vaccination before they even pushed the "play" button. The presence of a correlation between the viewing of the video and the behaviour (getting your child vaccinated) is therefore not evidence of a causal link between the two events. To establish causality more convincingly, it would have been necessary to ensure that there were no systematic differences between the parents of the two groups. One way to ensure the absence of such difference between parents who will be shown the video and those who will not is to randomly assign parents to one of the two groups. In doing so, the groups are somehow made equal except for the treatment, in this case the presentation of the video. Such a study is called a "randomised controlled trial" (RCT), whereas if there is no such randomisation, the study will be called "observational". In an RCT, the rate of vaccination in the two groups will be examined to see if the observed difference is consistent with what chance might produce. Indeed, it would be possible, and even quite expected for the vaccination rate not to be exactly identical in the two groups even if the video has no proven impact. Using appropriate statistical techniques, it can be established whether the observed difference between the two conditions is large enough to be deemed significant.

However, this study does not examine observational studies but only RCTs. In the case of descriptive norms, for example, it is purely by chance that people are confronted with a condition that highlights the normative (one could also say popular) or less frequent (i.e., unpopular) nature of a behaviour. Researchers then look at whether the subjects are aware of this normativity, of the popularity of the behaviour. In a second step, the researchers note the prevalence of intentions and behaviours in both conditions. The same approach prevails for prescriptive norms by informing people, for example, that a given behaviour is desired or condemned by individuals or reference groups. The results of no less than 21 studies and some 10,087 participants are unequivocal and attest to the effectiveness of the experimental manipulation of the norms and of their influence on intentions and behaviour. At the end of this analysis, 16 studies and 17 studies confirm that changing social norms modifies intentions and behaviour, respectively. 6 out of 10 people in the enhanced social norms condition score higher than someone randomly selected in the control condition. This is anything but trivial in the health domain.

It is clear that all health measures, including vaccination, are likely to be strongly influenced by the standards in place. This means, for example, that disclosure of information about the proportion of people who are motivated to be vaccinated is a crucial element in a vaccination campaign. In the face of the COVID-19 pandemic, many people were concerned about possible disaffection with vaccination. Psychologists were determined to rely on the strength of descriptive norms and the example set by those who were first vaccinated. Knowing, whether 20%, 50% or 80 % of the population supports vaccination is a crucial piece of information. There is a *bandwagoning* effect that can make a difference. Relying on people who are motivated, and therefore rather favourable to vaccination, will have an effect on the inclinations of others. These people are less likely to see the possible inconvenience of the injection as an insurmountable obstacle. This helps to spread an encouraging profile to a wider public, and the term is perfectly appropriate here – it gives more courage – to the less convinced citizens.

While descriptive norms are effective in promoting a behaviour that is already widely accepted, they can also be problematic when they correspond to courses of action that run counter to the desired direction. In the case of vaccination, the difficulty is not insignificant, given both the reluctance, and even resistance, expressed by part of the population and the ever-present temptation of the media to devote undue attention to problematic behaviour. In the same way that giving media space to a celebrity suicide increases the incidence of this type of behaviour, suggesting that a significant number of people question the wisdom of preventive measures or the usefulness of vaccination can reduce interest in it.

In an ingenious study conducted in February 2021 in the United States, i.e. at the very beginning of the vaccination campaign, researchers[8] showed their participants a website that supposedly designed to book appointments for vaccination in their county. Depending on the condition, subjects could see that 25% *versus* 75% of the time slots were still available, suggesting that many people (standard acceptance condition) *versus* few (standard hesitancy condition) wanted to be vaccinated. Furthermore, as they scrolled through the appointment page, some participants (high salience descriptive norm condition) noticed a change in status of one of the time slots. Specifically, those in the vaccine acceptance condition saw a slot change from blue (free slot) to red (reserved slot) status, while the reverse occurred for those in the vaccine hesitancy condition. Nothing in particular happened for the rest of the participants (low salience of the descriptive norm condition).

The data confirm that participants are more likely to perceive the situation as "normal" when few slots are still available than when many slots are still listed as available. More importantly for our purposes, they were less likely to delay, avoid or refuse vaccination when the norm emphasised acceptance rather than hesitancy, demonstrating the impact of descriptive norms. Better still, participants also demonstrated their sensitivity to the salience of the norm via the reservation dynamics presented to them. Thus, when people are confronted with only 25% of appointment slots already booked and see an additional slot become available before their eyes, they show even more vaccine hesitation. The opposite movement is seen when the displayed proportion of appointments is 75% and people see a live booking.

These results are in line with many studies that emphasise the importance of descriptive norms. In this respect, surveys of vaccine hesitancy confirm the crucial role of health care workers. The behaviour of doctors, nurses, pharmacists, etc., is a prime showcase.

But beyond this role as an example in the descriptive sense, the medical world also plays a major role as a "prescriber". This is also the case for the various sources that claim to have scientific expertise. One thinks of the WHO, the ECDC, government agencies, members of expert groups, consultants who parade around in the media. The same goes for political authorities. This time, we are obviously much closer to the notion of prescriptive norms associated with informal punishments or rewards.

PRESCRIPTIVE NORMS AND VACCINATION

Prescriptive norms are particularly useful when descriptive norms cannot be relied upon and imitation and spillover effects are expected. However, the sources of influence must have sufficient prestige and trust, which is easier to ensure when they have an almost horizontal relationship with the people who are expected to adopt the prescribed behaviour. In this respect, the data collected in the Motivation Barometer clearly establishes the importance of health care staff as a normative reference. Several surveys[9] also confirm that the proximity and legitimacy of these representatives of the medical world are quite different from those of the political authorities, with scientific experts being in an intermediate position. Yet the trust enjoyed by the medical world is not boundless. It is shaped by people's belief system and, singularly, by the way in which they exercise a trade-off between so-called allopathy (classical medicine) on the one hand and alternative medicines on the other.

While displaying the proportion of people vaccinated is an obvious way to inform the subjective norm, other strategies are sometimes mentioned. These include such basic interventions as badges or other signs displayed by the vaccinated. Some studies have in fact used these strategies. In one study,[10] health care workers in a Swiss hospital who had been vaccinated were asked to wear a badge saying "I have been vaccinated against the flu to protect you". Unvaccinated colleagues were asked to wear a mask during the epidemic season and a badge saying "I am wearing a mask to protect you". This manipulated both the prescriptive norm (with health care staff as "prescribers") and the descriptive norm (showing the number of vaccinated staff). In the year following the introduction of this measure, vaccination coverage rose to 37% from levels of 21–29% in the previous decade. Despite their clear benefits, there is a danger that the low number of people being vaccinated will become apparent. In the present case, one may also find oneself confronted with vaccine-hesitant staff, which increases the risk of vaccine hesitancy in this segment of the population as well.

NORM CONSISTENCY

During the COVID-19 pandemic, most people agreed that wearing a mask, keeping a safe distance between people and getting vaccinated were beneficial behaviours. In fact, a study[11] found that 80–90% of adults in the US considered wearing a mask to be an effective way to prevent the spread of the COVID-19 virus. Despite these impressive figures, only 50% of respondents said that they "always" or "most often" wore a mask when in close contact with others. It is of course good that people know what protective measures to take, but it is especially important that they actually do what the health authorities recommend!

In the field of social psychology, work on cognitive dissonance[12] has long focused on understanding those situations where there is a gap between a person's stated beliefs and their actual behaviour. There is widespread agreement that people should not waste precious drinking water or take precautions during sex to prevent STDs. Yet many people must admit that they leave their taps running for the duration of their ablutions or take showers for an inordinate amount of time. Ensuring that people do what they preach is at the heart of an approach known as 'induced hypocrisy'.[13] First, individuals are informed very explicitly about the intended behaviour, thus displaying their knowledge of what is considered desirable. In concrete terms, they are asked to write a text that develops their point of view or to record a video that includes their arguments. Afterwards, they are asked to point out any shortcomings or deficiencies on their part. Insofar as the revelation of this deviation undermines the sense of coherence that they intend to preserve, they are asked to correct the situation and adjust their subsequent conduct.

In an experiment[14] adopting this approach in the context of vaccination, participants began by evaluating a WHO video promoting protective measures, and in particular the wearing of masks. While some participants were then asked to give three reasons why the WHO health recommendations should be followed (the "Advocacy" condition), others were asked to write three sentences about situations in which they had not followed these recommendations (the "Failure" condition). In the induced hypocrisy condition, a third group performed both tasks. Finally, a control group was not subjected to either of the two requests. When recontacted one week later, participants in the induced hypocrisy condition were more likely than participants in the other conditions to comply with the health measures, whether it was wearing a mask, washing their hands or social distancing. They also reported more intentions to be vaccinated. Another relevant fact was that the least favourable condition was the failure condition. Although further work is needed to substantiate these findings, it seems prudent to refrain from misleading people if we want to encourage the intended behaviours.

As is the case in this study, work on induced hypocrisy tends to focus on situations where people do not object to the behaviours that are intended to be promoted.[15] This limitation is less problematic than it seems. Indeed, given the high level of acceptance of health measures, the real ambition is to get people who are convinced about the principles to act in accordance with them. In addition to the obvious direct effects, i.e. less spread of the virus and fewer infections, the social proof effect can play a role.

The driving force behind the effects of induced hypocrisy is not only the awareness of the inconsistency between one's behaviour and what one professes otherwise. The deviation from social norms also seems to be a determining factor.[16] While one can spontaneously think of social norms shared in society, the norms that will play the most crucial role are those associated to peers or, more broadly, to any relevant reference group. Hence the importance of how individuals perceive the social landscape. To which group(s) do they feel to belong, what are the key social identities on a chronic level or sometimes even in a given context?

ALTRUISM AND PARASITISM IN THE FIELD OF VACCINATION

As we have seen, reporting a social norm indicating that the expected behaviour, in this case vaccination, is popular among the population can have a knock-on effect. However, this involves a risk. Paradoxically, some people may feel that the high level of support for the vaccination campaign means that they do not need to follow suit. In other words, some people may take advantage of the fact that vaccination coverage is likely to reach sufficiently satisfactory levels to consider that their risk of contracting the disease is ultimately very limited and take advantage of this to avoid vaccination. This posture is problematic, even perverse. Indeed, people are perfectly entitled to oppose the vaccine for respectable reasons related to the possible risks at the time of vaccination and even more so in the long term, about which -admittedly- little is known. On the other hand, it is unpleasant that they should capitalise on the fact that others opt for vaccination and therefore incur possible negative consequences.

This "free-rider" behaviour is not nearly as rare as one might hope. While it is known that vaccination coverage does not need to reach 100% to be effective in combating a pandemic, the percentage that remains unvaccinated is thought to be mainly about people who cannot be vaccinated for reasons beyond their control. In fact, either because they have medical characteristics that make the vaccine inadvisable for them, or because they belong to a segment of the population for which it is not known whether it is possible to administer the vaccine, such as very young children, some people will in any case not be amenable to vaccination. It is therefore primarily for these people that we must be able to tolerate that coverage is not total. It is not only cynical, but also medically wrong to assume that it is safe to refuse vaccination when you are able to be vaccinated.

Going it alone or being a stowaway is not, by any means, a specificity of vaccination. In fact, this free-riding behaviour is at the heart of a stream of research on public goods and is part of the more general framework of game theory.[17] Work on the so-called "tragedy of the commons" provides information on people's incentives to contribute to the creation and maintenance of public goods (the "commons") and to the access of everyone to various goods and services.[18] The optimal situation occurs when everyone contributes equally to the common good. There are two ways in which people free-ride and parasitise the system by exploiting the cooperation of others and avoiding cooperation themselves. First, when the common good requires the investment of a critical threshold of people, the presence of enough contributors increases the temptation to refrain from making the effort, and all the more so because the exclusion of profiteers rarely occurs. Second, when people can draw on common goods that are somehow limited, the fact that resources are likely to be depleted quickly may lead some to draw beyond what is due to them (fishing is the best example in this regard). In general, the knowledge that enough members of the community are contributing to the common good, either by making an effort or by depriving themselves of a resource, fuels the temptation to free-ride. The data confirm that despite the initial existence of a strong willingness to cooperate among most, the difficulty of sanctioning free-riders eventually pushes many individuals to be less cooperative and to go it (slightly less) alone. More worryingly, experiments in the context of various infectious diseases show that the degree of parasitism increases as the rate of vaccination increases in the population.[19]

The COVID-19 pandemic is no exception to this sad reality, which is a major hurdle in the fight against the virus. Many people refuse to wear masks[20] or are reluctant to comply with requests for distancing[21] despite the proven effectiveness of these measures. In addition, the heterogeneity of the consequences of the disease for different groups of the population makes some people less likely to comply with the recommendations than others. For example, young people, who are less likely to suffer serious symptoms in the event of infection, are found to be less inclined to exercise caution. Even if the number of stowaways remains limited, the collective consequences can be dramatic.

How can this form of free riding be countered? One way out is through the negative emotional reactions that these postures elicit from cooperating people. Indeed, it seems that human beings are naturally inclined to identify and sanction parasites, whether through more diffuse norms or explicit sanctions. Vaccination is seen as a kind of social contract that people are supposed to respect. Thus, according to German researchers,[22] vaccination cannot be seen as a behaviour that is only in the interest of the individual, but must be considered in the context of the collective good. In other words, individuals are morally obliged to be vaccinated in order to protect others. If this is the prevailing view, then it should be observed that vaccination opens the way for gratitude and generosity on the part of vaccinated individuals towards other vaccinated individuals. This generosity should not be shown to those who choose not to be vaccinated, as they are perceived as not fulfilling the "social contract". This is precisely what these authors have shown through several experiments.

VACCINATION AND SOCIAL IDENTITY

In the midst of the COVID-19 pandemic, at a cordial family dinner, the issue of vaccination enters the discussion. Suddenly, the great-uncle with whom we had the most harmonious relations is transformed into a herald of resistance to the 'health dictatorship'. From that moment on, Richard is no longer the generous uncle, who does not fail to spoil his nieces and to shower his brothers with advice on the maintenance of their boiler, but he sees himself as the representative of a community, those who "are not sheep", who refuse to bend their backs in the face of what they perceive as arbitrary decisions from the authorities. This community manifests itself in the Facebook group "Citizens wake up!", whose posts he religiously reads and which he does not fail to enrich with videos or articles discovered in the course of his research. The family discussion turns into a pugilism between two camps. On one side of the barricades, Richard and his daughter-in-law Sarah also a member of this group, and on the other, the rest of the family, people who see themselves as "rational", concerned about the health of others and their loved ones, and who give credence to the discourse of the authorities and the academic experts who advise them. This latter group has also changed their "costume": when the discussion gets heated, they have abandoned their role as father, mother, brother, daughter, but see themselves as representatives of a larger community, as "realists" who "trust science", etc. Some also have their own groups on social networks, where they share the latest claims of this or that anti-vaccination guru with mocking smileys.

The description of this discussion, which may awaken some memories, resonates with an idea developed in the framework of social identity theory (SIT).[23] According to this theory, the way we define ourselves varies according to the context. And, particularly in certain contexts, we see ourselves as individuals, distinct from other individuals. This definition of self is what SIT calls personal identity. Our behaviour is then guided by the traits and characteristics that differentiate us from other individuals. For example, Richard defines himself as an 'uncle' in this context and being "generous" is an important characteristic for him.

In other contexts, on the other hand, individuals would define themselves as members of a community and their individual identity would hardly be in the foreground. It is the way in which they perceive their group (ingroup) in relation to other groups (outgroups) that would guide their conduct. In such situations, individuals would tend to see themselves as interchangeable members of the same group, to "depersonalise" themselves. The #MeToo *hashtag*, which flourished in the wake of the Harvey Weinstein scandal, was a way for the Internet users who wrote it to show that, beyond their singular experiences, they shared a common belonging through their experiences of sexual harassment or sexual assault. In such "intergroup" situations, the outgroup (e.g. "pigs") will be perceived as essentially, and profoundly, different from the ingroup. In the context of vaccination, figures such as "elites", "mainstream media" or "Big Pharma" may have played this role.

This shift from a personal to a social identity can be triggered by many factors. But it is clear that the social and political context is likely to make some identities more relevant or salient. Being "infected", "at risk", "confined", "out of work" are states that shape our individual behaviour. We need to take them into account in order to act in the most appropriate way possible. In the context of a pandemic, these characteristics can suddenly become the basis of social identities and guide coordinated behaviour within groups that define themselves in this way, which then becomes a matter for *collective action*.

How do social identities influence behaviour? According to social identity theory, individuals place a *value on* this identity: it could be more or less favourable. For example, in India, the identity of *Dalit* "Untouchables" may be perceived as negative in comparison with that of valued castes, such as *Brahmins* or *Kshatriyas*. In the context of COVID-19 vaccination, being unvaccinated may have been a source of negative identity, as it restricted access to certain activities (due to vulnerability to COVID-19 or to restrictions imposed by the authorities, through the "health pass" and other equivalent measures).

In this regard, one should note that during the COVID-19 pandemic, vaccinated people as well as those guided by some social identity made salient by the health situation showed particularly negative attitudes towards unvaccinated people. In a study conducted from December 2021 to January 2022, Danish researchers[24] asked respondents from 21 countries how unhappy they would be if a member of their family married a non-vaccinated person. The results were clear: the dissatisfaction would be considerable! It was on average 2.5 times more than if the spouse in question was an immigrant, a common target of prejudice. While there may be good reasons for these attitudes, the unvaccinated could therefore legitimately feel rejected by the vaccinated.

In the eyes of many people, some anti-vaxxers have gone overboard in wearing the yellow star to highlight the fact that they are stigmatised. Yet individuals should be motivated to develop a positive identity. This involves making favourable comparisons with other groups, which is a function of *social differentiation*. In the above example, stereotypes play this role. "We", say the pro-vaxxers, are "rational" while they "have been brainwashed". "We", say the anti-vaxxers, are "resistants" (mobilising another World War II analogy) who refuse to bow to health dictatorship and fight against the deprivation of our freedoms, unlike these "sheep".

Research on vaccine hesitancy demonstrates the importance of these identity processes. For example, in a 2018 study, an Australian team[25] interviewed parents who refused or were reluctant to vaccinate their children. These interviews showed a segmentation of their social environment into two categories, namely families who vaccinate and those who do not. The former would be "unhealthy" while the latter would be "healthy", thus articulating a comparison favourable to the in-group. Many observations (which may be confirmation bias, see above) support this worldview: while the unvaccinated would be perfectly healthy, say the parents, the vaccinated would be riddled with all sorts of ailments (supposedly, because their "natural immunity" could hardly develop). The outgroup is seen to adopt a whole range of unhealthy practices: eating frozen food, consuming medication without "listening to their bodies". Some see themselves as "enlightened" elites and distinguish themselves from "sheep" who do not even realise that there is an alternative to their unhealthy lifestyle.

These identity processes are fed by exchanges with other members of the group, particularly online or during public meetings or events. These interactions can have several effects. On the one hand, they underline that they are not alone, that their identity is shared. This confers a sense of power, of strength in numbers, which will facilitate the expression of positions that may seem contrary to the dominant norm in society. Moreover, these interactions confront members with the discourses of "leaders" or "influencers" who offer a reading of the social context, the conflicts that organise this context, and the identities in which they are inserted. Thus, when some of them describe the pandemic as an invention based on a "pseudovirus" and vaccination as a "global deception" organised by Bill Gates, they offer a reading of the health situation that points to identifiable enemies and articulates these with a favourable identity. Indeed, isn't it brave to resist mischievous businessmen ready to sacrifice the weakest in order to line their pockets?

This approach invites us to consider vaccine hesitancy in the light of shifting identities, the content of which may vary according to the evolution of the social context. Rather than seeing this posture as a trait firmly anchored in the psyche of individuals, we need to look at the contextual factors likely to favour this type of positioning. For example, in France, the opposition between the "haves" and the "have-nots" is particularly vivid and played an important role in the structuring of the yellow vests movement,[26] fuelled by a vision of power "on the payroll of the rich". The anti-vax stance also feeds on this opposition, which was rekindled by the pandemic, particularly when the lockdown affected the most disadvantaged, confined to cramped housing outside urban areas, to a much greater extent. Resentments accumulated in this first phase of the pandemic (in the absence of a vaccine) and identities could be grafted onto these resentments. Anti-vaccinism then appeared as an opposition to the "system".

The "us/them" categorisation is not just about distinguishing ourselves from others in a positive way. By identifying an outgroup and attributing a range of traits, characteristics and values to it ("Who we are not"), we can identify who *we* are. Nothing is more mobilising than knowing who our "enemy" is. An American study[27] illustrates this point impressively. The authors analysed thousands of messages (*tweets* and Facebook posts) from political figures and media outlets clearly identified by their political affiliation (Democrat or Republican). They found that messages naming members of the opposite party were shared much more widely on the networks than those naming one's own party. This factor was even more predictive of the sharing than was the emotional tone of the message.

Just as vaccine-averse parents in Australia pitted "healthy" against "unhealthy" people, a similar dynamic characterises the identities associated with vaccination. From the perspective of those who embrace vaccination, the hesitant are seen as a foil. In an international study,[28] vaccinated people saw non-vaccinated as untrustworthy and unintelligent. This dynamic rests on the use of a category that refers to a perceived homogeneous outgroup. However, it is clear that the individuals and groups designated in this way can have very diverse positions with regard to vaccination. By grouping them in the same category, "anti-vaxxers", we come to see them all as hostile to the very principle of vaccination, as reactionary obscurantists in relation to whom the ingroup can define itself as "enlightened".

A French study[29] examined the representation of people designated as anti-vaxxers in the French press (between 1990 and 2017), on Twitter (in 2016) and on websites challenging at least one vaccine recommendation. It appears that, predominantly, the term "anti-vax" carries a negative connotation. Anti-vaxxers come across as cognitively limited and unable to think rationally. Presumably, this is due to the grip of emotions and "ideologies". Worse, anti-vaxxers would be the vectors of a social movement aiming to spread their irrational beliefs through "propaganda". As to "pro-vaxxers", they see science as the supreme embodiment of rationality, an activity that should not be subordinated to emotions, religions or ideologies. Through this portrayal, anti-vaxxers are perceived as a threat not only to a specific public health practice (vaccination), but to a central value, the reliability of *science*. Given the emblematic nature of this view of the anti-vax posture, the authors of this study show that it also emerges in other debates, unrelated to vaccination. For example, in a Twitter debate on osteopathy, the latter was described as a "shitty" practice and linked to anti-vaxxers.

In this respect, this study reveals a paradoxical reversal: this denigrating label leads many actors who are critical of vaccination to distinguish themselves from it. They present themselves, for example, as favourable to "vaccine freedom" and sometimes explicitly distinguish themselves from anti-vaxxers, even presenting themselves as "moderate" "neither in favour nor against the vaccine". By adopting a disparaging view of antivaxxers, they can thus appear all the more credible. In doing so, these critical vaccine actors, far from conforming to the above stereotypes, also claim to be scientific. Turning the tables they see themselves as victims of a sectarian practice of science. They would indeed be the target of "fatwas", "crusades", and "papal bulls" (terms from the religious register, thus). They would use science in a "critical" and independent way (suggesting that the "pro-vaxxers" are under the influence of financial interests). Through this game of mirrors, we see how two identities are constructed in opposition with both claiming to be science-driven and stigmatising their nemesis.

SOCIAL IDENTITY AND TRUST

In the previous chapter, we examined the role of trust in vaccination attitudes. Trust in the actors of vaccination is likely to vary according to the social insertion of individuals and their social identity. To the extent that the ethnic, cultural, gender, sexual orientation groups that make up a society have had diverse experiences with some of these actors, these can of course play a role in the trust felt towards them and, when a vaccination campaign is implemented, influence vaccine uptake. For example, in the United States, African Americans are notoriously less enthusiastic about vaccination than European Americans. In view of the discriminatory nature of the American health system and considering the many abuses committed against African American populations in the name of medicine (forced sterilisations, unscrupulous pharmaceutical trials, discrimination in the quality of treatment, etc.), this is hardly surprising.

Individuals or communities are more or less distant from primary care. This reality can be explained by an array of factors such as financial, geographical (medical deserts), administrative, linguistic or psychological (e.g., underestimation of risk) barriers. Unsurprisingly, confidence is lower among those people and communities that are further away from the health system. For example, a study conducted in 2021 among young "racialised" people in the Brussels neighbourhood of Molenbeek found a lack of enthusiasm for vaccination against COVID-19. This confirms the data on the very low vaccination coverage in this area. If these young people do not wish to be vaccinated, it is not because they do not have confidence in the vaccine itself. Rather, some mention a distrust of hospitals and doctors, whom they see as preoccupied mainly with financial concerns: "you go to the hospital and you see a doctor, everything is fine . . . then two weeks later you get the bill, there, with lines you didn't ask for. But you still have to pay." (p. 3)[30] Some respondents also mentioned having been confronted with racist discourse when they went to the hospital. Medical actors come across as part of a larger system that seeks to monitor, control, and even punish patients or members of their community. From this perspective, vaccine refusal is only the end of a long chain that originates in a mistrust of all institutions.

However, while trust in authorities may play a positive role in attitudes towards vaccination, this is not always the case. For example, in a study conducted in the United States in the summer of 2020,[31] a negative relationship emerged between trust in government and intention to vaccinate against COVID-19 in several US cities. This is because opposition to vaccination has been mobilised for political purposes by the Trump administration, which has deployed it as a marker of a partisan (in this case, Republican) identity. This example illustrates the importance that social identity plays in trust. We trust others to the extent that we consider that they share a common group membership with us. This can be very general and based, for example, on common values (benevolence, concern for future generations, etc.). In order to induce such a feeling, it is important that the authorities can be seen to be *representative of the* whole population to which they are addressing themselves. If they seem disconnected from the people, if they are like disembodied elites whose concerns are not our own, they are unlikely to generate trust, as they will be perceived as an outgroup. In the end, support for a public health policy depends less on the content of the message than on the affiliation of the person proposing it. For example, researchers[32] presented different COVID-related policies to respondents from seven different countries. The recommendations were presented either as coming from "liberal" (i.e. "left-wing") groups, "conservative" groups, or both, or from experts. The political orientation of the subjects was also assessed. Respondents liked a policy more if it came from their own political group than from the opposite group. Thus, political affiliations have a *polarising* effect. In contrast, experts had a "depolarising" effect: when a policy was supported by experts, there was more support for it, regardless of its political orientation. This effect is explained by trust: one trusts more a source categorised as ingroup.[33] This is true of like-minded politicians, but also of like-minded scientists if we value science and expertise. These elements can, as we have seen, be strong identity markers in a pandemic context.

Of course, other identity markers can play an important role. In the Belgian context, for example, decisions on the management of the COVID-19 crisis were taken by an assembly of political representatives from different levels of government (federal, regional, etc.). At the end of their meetings, the head of the federal government communicated the decisions on prime time television with the heads of the country's regional/community governments, most of them men, all of them "white" and over 40 years old. Perhaps this was not the ideal configuration to convince those who did not fit these profiles to follow the proposed measures. In an US study,[34] pro-vaccination content was presented to Christians. These messages were presented in the form of a short biography of the director of the National Institute of Health (NIH), a video interview with him and a text. In a control condition, the messages focused solely on public health issues. In an experimental condition, the director's Christian faith was emphasised. In this condition, respondents showed greater trust in the expert, which was reflected in a higher intention to be vaccinated.

CONFORMITY AND SOCIAL IDENTITY

The above leads us back to the role of social norms in behaviour. In light of the social identity approach, conformity is rooted in the way individuals perceive themselves in terms of their identity. In a study that illustrates this point admirably,[35] the researchers drew on the Autokinetic Effect paradigm, famous in social psychology and originally introduced by Sherif[36] to study individual conformity. Sherif had invited participants to estimate the movement of a bright spot in a perfectly dark room. In this situation, any apparent motion actually results from a perfect an optical illusion. While, unsurprisingly, estimates varied significantly from person to person in the single-person condition, a rapid convergence occurred when several people performed the exercise together. According to Sherif, this pattern attests to the strong need for people to agree if they are convinced that there is a single reality.

In the more social version, the experiment was conducted with six people, only three of whom were naive. The others, the experimenter's confederates were each asked to take notes of the responses of one of the three naive participants. The task consisted of 25 estimates given in turn, starting with the naive followed by the confederates. The specific task of the latter was to add 5 cm to the first three estimates provided by "their" *alter ego* and then to stay within 2 cm of their third response. The assumption was that this initial gap in estimates would prevent convergence. To certify the role of social affiliations on the formation and adoption of norms, three conditions were used to manipulate the degree of salience of the two entities. In addition to a first condition in which there was no mention of a distinction between people (implicit condition), another condition (category condition) explicitly mentioned the existence of two categories of subjects during the experiment. Finally, in a last condition, each member of two entities was addressed, always naming the group to which they belonged (group condition). It was found that, in the "implicit" condition, the naive participants showed quite different responses from those of the accomplices, but more importantly, that this tendency became more pronounced as the memberships became more palpable (category and group respectively).

Self-categorisation theory,[37] which developed from social identity theory, helps to explain these results. According to this theory, when individuals define themselves according to a specific collective belonging, they tend to seek a consensus with the members of this social category to elaborate a shared worldview. But which worldview, which norms will be favoured? According to this theory, one will conform to the most "prototypical" point of view of the group, which itself depends on the comparison with the outgroup. It is the latter's opinion that best differentiates the ingroup. In the study reported here, the confederates were the outgroup and thus, by contrast, defined the ingroup 'norm' to which naive participants conformed.

NORMS AND POLARISATION

A phenomenon that is particularly striking in the COVID-19 vaccination debate is not in itself new, but has taken on a new dimension with the advent of social networks. It is what social psychologists call "group polarisation". A little background information is helpful in this regard.

If, as we saw in the previous chapter, we prefer to expose ourselves to information that is consistent with our attitudes, we also choose to interact with people who are similar to us – this is called "homophily". By bringing together people who are similar and who have a predilection for information that confirms their pre-existing attitudes, don't social networks act as sounding boards? Indeed, every time someone puts forward an idea, it can be assumed that others, with similar views, simply repeat and reinforce it by sharing content that echoes their beliefs. This type of dynamic can produce group polarisation[38]: everyone is reinforced in their position and develops more and more extreme attitudes.

Here again, self-categorisation theory helps to shed light on this phenomenon.[39] As we have just seen, this approach assumes that the "norm" of the ingroup corresponds to the position deemed "prototypical" of the group. But this prototype is likely to be more extreme than the average position of the group members. For example, if you put environmental activists together, a more radical member may seem more "representative" of the group, because his position allows him to be more clearly distinguished from relevant out-groups (e.g., supporters of fossil fuel extraction). By seeking to conform to this prototype, group members in turn radicalise their position, which corresponds to the polarisation dynamic.

According to this explanation, if we are influenced by what is said in the "network", it is because we define ourselves as members of the same group as those who are there with us. When we identify with a group, it becomes the source of our outlook on reality and we seek to be in consonance with its other members. The information exchanged then serves to identify the "prototypical" position of our group.

An Italian team[40] tested the hypothesis of polarisation in relation to the topic of vaccination. The authors studied Facebook users discussing vaccination. For each person, their vaccination tendency was estimated according to the content shared (pro- or anti-vaccine) and the tendencies of the people with whom they interacted (their "network"). In line with the homophily hypothesis, there is a propensity to be connected to like-minded people. The research also looked at the dissemination of information and found that, on Facebook in particular, users tend to receive information that conforms to their pre-existing attitudes. Gradually, this selective exposure to information that is consistent with their attitudes creates real "communities" characterised by a specific orientation towards vaccination.

While these results may seem worrying, they need to be qualified because they relate only to the dissemination of information and not to the actual attitudes or beliefs of users. Another large-scale study[41] examined the temporal evolution of attitudes towards COVID-19 vaccination among US citizens in 2021 as a function of exposure to misinformation. The authors assessed three types of variables. First, exposure to misinformation about COVID-19, by asking their subjects whether they had heard of various fake news about the virus; second, adherence to false beliefs about vaccination (and related to these fake news); and third, their attitudes towards COVID-19 vaccination. As this study was conducted in three successive waves (longitudinal study) with the same individuals, it allows causal relationships to be established more convincingly than a cross-sectional study and several questions to be answered.

Firstly, is there a polarisation of attitudes over time? The answer is yes (see the horizontal arrows linking attitudes between the three waves in the lower part of Figure 3.1).

Secondly, does exposure to misinformation lead to even more exposure later on? The answer is also yes, which confirms the resonance box hypothesis (see horizontal arrows in the upper part of Figure 3.1).

Thirdly, do false beliefs also reinforce themselves (see the horizontal arrows in the middle section of Figure 3.1)?

More specifically, the study shows that the strengthening of attitudes is explained by several beliefs. People who are favourable to vaccination tend to adhere less and less to fake news, which makes them even more favourable to vaccination. Conversely, people who hold unfounded beliefs about vaccination become less and less supportive (see arrows from "adherence" to "attitude").

So far, the "dangerous echo chamber" narrative is supported. However, the results do not show an effect of exposure to misinformation on adherence or attitudes. This study also fails to establish a selective information effect based on attitudes or adherence (see Chapter 2): prior attitudes do not appear to condition subsequent exposure. If there is selective exposure, it is of a different nature: having been

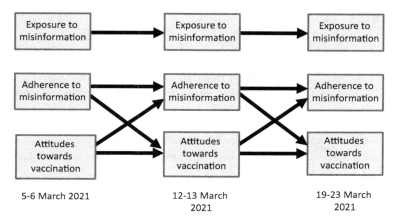

Figure 3.1 Results of Xu *et al.* (2022)

exposed to certain information makes us more likely to be exposed to the same type of information later. These results, which are somewhat surprising compared to the studies mentioned above, can be explained by several factors. One is that this study was conducted at a time when the COVID-19 vaccination was in the news. The subjects were therefore confronted with a great deal of information on the subject, which may have limited the impact of misinformation. In addition, unlike the laboratory studies discussed above, the effect of exposure to misinformation was assessed one week later, and thus may have dissipated.

Finally, the study does not answer an obvious question: how can we explain that subjects develop unfounded beliefs about vaccination if not through exposure to them? One answer is that while beliefs drive attitudes, the reverse is also true. In this study, it was found that as attitudes changed, subjects increasingly held beliefs that were consistent with their attitudes. It is as if, in the set of information they were confronted with, subjects chose to adhere to those that allowed them to reinforce their attitudes, a phenomenon that is part of motivated reasoning (see Chapter 2).

NOTES

1 Yzerbyt, V., & Klein, O. (2023). *Psychologie Sociale* [Psychologie Sociale]. 2nd Ed. Louvain-la-Neuve, Belgium: De Boeck.

2 Cialdini, R. B. (2006). *Influence: The psychology of persuasion*. New York: Harper.

3 Newcomb, T. M. (1943). *Personality and social change; attitude formation in a student community*. New York: Dryden Press.

4 Cialdini, R. B. (2006). *Op. cit.*

5 Bandura, A. (1965). Influence of models' reinforcement contingencies on the acquisition of imitative responses. *Journal of Personality and Social Psychology*, 1(6), 589–595.

6 Phillips, D. P. (1974). The influence of suggestion on suicide: Substantive and theoretical implications of the Werther effect. *American Sociological Review*, 39(3), 340–354.

7 Sheeran, P., Maki, A., Montanaro, E., Avishai-Yitshak, A., Bryan, A., Klein, W. M. P., Miles, E., & Rothman, A. J. (2016). The impact of changing attitudes, norms, and self-efficacy on health-related intentions and behavior: A meta-analysis. *Health Psychology*, 35(11), 1178–1188.

8 Ryoo, Y., & Kim, W. (2021). Using descriptive and injunctive norms to encourage COVID-19 social distancing and vaccinations. *Health Communication*, 1–10.

9 Goubert, L., Klein, O., Luminet, O., Morbée, S., Schmitz, M., Van den Bergh, O., Van Oost, P., Vansteenkiste, M., Yzerbyt, V., & Waterschoot, J. (2022). *Motivation, well-being and attitudes towards vaccination in the time of the omicron. Motivation Barometer Report*, 39. Belgium: Ghent University. https://motivationbarometer.com/en/portfolio-item/rapport-39-motivatie-welbevinden-en-vaccinatie-attitudes-in-omikron-tijden/.

10 Iten, A., Bonfillon, C., Boymond, S., Siegrist, C.-A., & Pittet, D. (2015). Improving vaccination against seasonal influenza among healthcare workers, 1994–2015. *Antimicrobial Resistance and Infection Control*, 4(1), 17.

11 Darling, J., Thomas, K., Kapteyn, A., Theys, N., & Cassil, A. (2021). *Most U.S. adults wear masks – inconsistently*. Understanding Coronavirus in America Tracking Survey, USC Schaeffer Center for Health Policy and Economics. https://healthpolicy.usc.edu/evidence-base/most-u-s-adults-wear-masks-inconsistently.

12 Festinger, L. (1957). *A theory of cognitive dissonance*. Vol. 2. Stanford: Stanford University Press.

13 Aronson, E., Fried, C., & Stone, J. (1991). Overcoming denial and increasing the intention to use condoms through the induction of hypocrisy. *American Journal of Public Health, 81*(12), 1636–1638.

14 Pearce, L., & Cooper, J. (2021). Fostering COVID-19 safe behaviors using cognitive dissonance. *Basic and Applied Social Psychology, 42*(5), 267–282.

15 For example: Fointiat, V., Priolo, D., Saint-Bauzel, R., & Milhabet, I. (2013). Justifying our transgressions to reduce our hypocrisy? Induced hypocrisy and the identification of transgressions. *International Journal of Social Psychology, 26*(4), 49–78.

16 Priolo, D., Pelt, A., Bauzel, R. S., Rubens, L., Voisin, D., & Fointiat, V. (2019). Three decades of research on induced hypocrisy: A meta-analysis. *Personality and Social Psychology Bulletin, 45*(12), 1681–1701.

17 Yong, J. C., & Choy, B. K. C. (2021). Noncompliance with safety guidelines as a free-riding strategy: An evolutionary game-theoretic approach to cooperation during the COVID-19 pandemic. *Frontiers in Psychology, 12.*

18 For example: Hardin, G. (1968). The tragedy of the commons: The population problem has no technical solution; it requires a fundamental extension in morality. *Science, 162*(3859), 1243–1248.

19 Ibuka, Y., Li, M., Vietri, J., Chapman, G. B., & Galvani, A. P. (2014). Free-riding behavior in vaccination decisions: An experimental study. *PLOS One, 9*(1), e87164.

20 Kramer, S. (2020). *More Americans say they are regularly wearing masks in stores and other businesses.* Pew Research Center. www.pewresearch.org/fact-tank/2020/08/27/more-americans-say-they-are-regularly-wearing-masks-in-stores-and-other-businesses.

21 Murphy, K., Williamson, H., Sargeant, E., & McCarthy, M. (2020). Why people comply with COVID-19 social distancing restrictions: Self-interest or duty? *Australian & New Zealand Journal of Criminology, 53*(4), 477–496.

22 Korn, L., Böhm, R., Meier, N. W., & Betsch, C. (2020). Vaccination as a social contract. *Proceedings of the National Academy of Sciences, 117*(26), 14890–14899.

23 Tajfel, H., & Turner, J. C. (1986). The social identity theory of intergroup behavior. In Worchel, S., & Austin, W. G. (Eds.), *Psychology of intergroup relations* (pp. 7–24). Chicago: Nelson Hall.

24 Bor, A., Jørgensen, F., & Petersen, M. B. (2022). Discriminatory attitudes against the unvaccinated during a global pandemic. *Nature, 613,* 704–711.

25 Attwell, K., Smith, D. T., & Ward, P. R. (2018). 'The unhealthy other': How vaccine-rejecting parents construct the vaccinating mainstream. *Vaccine, 36*(12), 1621–1626.

26 Jetten, J., Mols, F., & Selvanathan, H. P. (2020). How economic inequality fuels the rise and persistence of the yellow vest movement. *International Review of Social Psychology*, 33(1).

27 Rathje, S., Van Bavel, J. J., & van der Linden, S. (2021). Out-group animosity drives engagement on social media. *Proceedings of the National Academy of Sciences*, 118(26), e2024292118.

28 Bor, A. *et al.* (2022). *Op. cit.*

29 Ward, J. K., Guille-Escuret, P., & Alapetite, C. (2019). Les «antivaccins», figure de l'anti-science [The antivaxx-embodiment of opposition to science]. *Déviance et Société*, 43(2), 221–251.

30 Maes, R. (2021). La spirale de la disaffiliation [The spiral of disaffiliation]. *La Revue Nouvelle*, 6(6), 2–5.

31 Trent, M., Seale, H., Chughtai, A. A., Salmon, D., & MacIntyre, C. R. (2022). Trust in government, intention to vaccinate and COVID-19 vaccine hesitancy: A comparative survey of five large cities in the United States, United Kingdom, and Australia. *Vaccine*, 40(17), 2498–2505.

32 Flores, A., Cole, J. C., Dickert, S., Eom, K., Jiga-Boy, G. M., Kogut, T., Loria, R., Mayorga, M., Pedersen, E. J., Pereira, B., Rubaltelli, E., Sherman, D. K., Slovic, P., Västfjäll, D., & Van Boven, L. (2022). Politicians polarize and experts depolarize public support for COVID-19 management policies across countries. *Proceedings of the National Academy of Sciences*, 119(3), e2117543119.

33 Cole, J. C., Flores, A., Jiga-Boy, G. M., Klein, O., Sherman, D. K., & Van Boven, L. (2023). Party over pandemic: Polarized trust in political leaders and experts explains public support for COVID-19 policies. *Group Processes & Intergroup Relations*, 26(7), 1611–1640.

34 Chu, J., Pink, S. L., & Willer, R. (2021). Religious identity cues increase vaccination intentions and trust in medical experts among American Christians. *Proceedings of the National Academy of Sciences*, 118(49), e2106481118.

35 Abrams, D., Wetherell, M., Cochrane, S., Hogg, M. A., & Turner, J. C. (1990). Knowing what to think by knowing who you are: Self-categorization and the nature of norm formation, conformity and group polarization. *The British Journal of Social Psychology*, 29(2), 97–119.

36 Sherif, M. (1936). *The psychology of social norms*. Oxford: Harper.

37 Turner, J. C., Hogg, M. A., Oakes, P., Reicher, S., & Wetherell, M. S. (1987). *Rediscovering the social group: A self-categorization theory*. Oxford: Blackwell.

38 Moscovici, S., & Zavalloni, M. (1969). The group as a polarizer of attitudes. *Journal of Personality and Social Psychology*, 12(2), 125.

39 McGarty, C., Turner, J. C., Hogg, M. A., David, B., & Wetherell, M. S. (1992). Group polarization as conformity to the prototypical group member. *British Journal of Social Psychology*, 31(1), 119.

40 Cinelli, M., De Francisci Morales, G., Galeazzi, A., Quattrociocchi, W., & Starnini, M. (2021). The echo chamber effect on social media. *Proceedings of the National Academy of Sciences of the United States of America*, 118(9), e2023301118.

41 Xu, S., Coman, I. A., Yamamoto, M., & Najera, C. J. (2022). Exposure effects or confirmation bias? Examining reciprocal dynamics of misinformation, misperceptions, and attitudes toward COVID-19 vaccines. *Health Communication*, 38(10), 111.

4

VACCINATION AND SOCIAL THOUGHT

The term "infodemic", which takes up the metaphor of an epidemic, suggests that we are overwhelmed by information, true or false. In order to penetrate people's discourse and influence their behaviour, this information must ultimately behave like a virus. It must be integrated into more elaborate forms of thought, produced and circulated within social groups. This is what Rouquette calls "social thought".[1] Here we will consider three forms, namely social representations, rumours, and conspiracy theories. In fact, even if research on the effects of misinformation and disinformation on vaccination does not necessarily call upon these concepts, most of the examples encountered in this type of work fit easily into these forms of social thought.

SOCIAL REPRESENTATIONS AND VACCINATION

For a long time, science was seen as an activity reserved for "specialists", with recognised expertise and high level degrees, who exchanged information in restricted circles and published mainly for their peers. With the development of the "public sphere" around the end of the 18th century, from the press to Wikipedia, YouTube and social networks, this knowledge has escaped from these limited

DOI: 10.4324/9781032665429-5

circles and has begun to be transmitted to the average person. In the process, however, it has been transformed, some would say altered, triturated and even abused. In the field of 'exact' sciences, the theory of relativity and that of natural selection are not within everyone's reach. The same is true in the social sciences when it comes to understanding marxism or psychoanalysis.

This transmission is particularly interesting to observe when new scientific knowledge emerges that is likely to transform our lives in a more or less radical way. Unsurprisingly, the general public is particularly keen to learn about knowledge that could influence their well-being or health. Think of genetically modified organisms, subliminal images, climate change or even microwaves, all of which require knowledge far beyond that of a person with a secondary or even higher education in a field not directly related to the phenomenon at hand.

The way expert knowledge becomes lay knowledge and is transmitted within a society is at the heart of the theory of social representations developed by Serge Moscovici.[2] Moscovici was initially interested in psychoanalysis and how elements of this theory were assimilated within society. According to Moscovici, a form of "lay science" is developed to make sense of these unknown realities. To do so, this lay science integrates elements from "expert knowledge" but that are not necessarily sufficient to understand these new realities. It is a question of "filling in the gaps" by calling on knowledge that has already been assimilated. This integration is all the more important because, in order to make sense of the phenomena to which these innovations refer, whether they are conceptual or material in nature, we cannot rely solely on direct observation. Who has ever seen the cystic fibrosis gene? Who has come across the libido? Who has observed the SARS-CoV2 virus? Our experience of these realities or of the mechanisms involved can often only be indirect. We must therefore 'recycle' expert knowledge to make sense of these non-directly observable realities.

It is during this process that social representations intervene, which can be defined as "systems of opinions, knowledge and beliefs specific to a culture or group in relation to an object in the social environment".[3] Social representations concern the way in which a community will appropriate expert knowledge, most often through the press or the media. While the "vertical" dimension (from the "experts" or the "media" to the public) is crucial, these social representations also unfold through communication within the communities concerned, this time in a horizontal manner.

According to Moscovici, expert knowledge is produced by a style of thinking which he describes as "formal", acquired through instruction and which operates by logical reasoning and by confrontation with reality. The "natural" style of thinking, on the other hand, does not require any training but is developed through our interactions, drawing its validity from its social value, from its capacity to create social links. To understand this distinction in the context of vaccination, let us consider the case of Dr. Van Metheal. In his practice, he considers the value of a vaccine in terms of its effectiveness, i.e. its ability to reduce the risk of infection accompanied by symptoms. This percentage would have to be established by a controlled study. When he plays golf with his club members, his knowledge of the world of vaccination, and of the vaccine, takes on a different value. It allows him to show off and establish his social status in relation to his friends, doctors as well as others. The value of a vaccine is then measured by the degree to which it allows Dr. Van Metheal to play to the gallery with his knowledge of it (there is nothing like messenger RNA vaccines to do this). The same person can thus use two different ways of thinking to evoke the same phenomenon. This social function of knowledge can lead to the valorisation of knowledge because it is shared and therefore allows integration into the community. So, let's imagine ourselves in the shoes of a 16-year-old whose parents think that the COVID-19 RNA vaccine will "change their DNA". It is undoubtedly tempting to conform to this social representation, promoted in this family circle, simply because it is the subject of a consensus and helps to strengthen the social bond. It will therefore take all the more determination for Aaron Williams, a New York teenager of this age, to escape his parents' grip and get vaccinated anyway.[4]

What determines the transition from one form of thinking to the other? According to Moscovici, we think through two distinct cognitive systems. The first system, which he calls "operative", functions by associations ("COVID-19 is like the flu"), inclusion ("by refusing the health dictatorship, you are a resistant"), discrimination ("vaccines are artificial, vitamins are natural"), and so forth. The second, which he calls "metasystem", controls the functioning of this first system according to criteria and rules that depend on the context. In a context where scientific accuracy is the order of the day, this metasystem can produce a formal style, whereas it could lead to a "natural style" if it allows the production of simple representations that can be used to obtain a desired behaviour from a hurried or busy audience at little cost.

Social representations are *social* not only because they are manifested within a community but also, and above all, because they are exchanged between individuals through social interactions. By conversing about an object, people validate their mutual representations of that object. What was only a thought becomes a reality from the point of view of the partners in the conversation. Potentially far-fetched ideas can thus appear as less and less contestable realities as they are exchanged and validated by those who converse about them.

Two mechanisms play an essential role in this transition from expert to layman, from the unknown to the familiar. *Objectification* consists in making the abstract concrete through a process of reification. It involves transforming vague beliefs or information into certainties, corresponding to a reality independent of the one who bears it and often to concrete images. For example, in the case of psychoanalysis, the concept of "complex" was sometimes perceived as a "tumour". The idea that messenger RNA vaccines inject "the virus" or "the disease" is to transform an unknown or poorly understood concept into a reality that seems more tangible. Objectification is also achieved by *embodying* the risks supposedly posed by the vaccine in concrete people. For example, a person will be shown as having become (supposedly) severely disabled following an injection. This process of objectification facilitates communication about the object of the representation. Indeed, in most social contexts, pharmacovigilance statistics are much less easy (and interesting) to communicate than striking cases of adverse effects (real or supposed), especially if they are directly visible and based on moving testimonies. In some groups, the vaccine can be seen as the materialisation of certain social relationships: between the state and citizens, between technology and the body, between modern medicine and the individual, etc. Thanks to its capacity to crystallise these social relations, which are *a priori* different, the vaccine offers an ideal support for objectification. The fact that it serves to inject a substance that comes from outside, and is therefore a mediator between two distinct spaces, is a fundamental explanatory factor. Through objectification, the perception of the vaccine becomes part of global representations of society, which it actualises in a concrete way.

The second mechanism, *anchoring*, consists in interpreting a still unknown object with the help of familiar categories. Thus, Moscovici notes that, for many French people, the figure of the psychoanalyst (poorly known at the time) is associated with that of the priest (well known). Social representations thus operate by integrating unknown elements into a repertoire of ordinary and well-mastered knowledge. To make sense of vaccination, it can of course be anchored in easily understandable representations, such as war metaphors (for example, seeing the cells of the immune system as an 'army' training to fight the virus). More generally, vaccination can be seen as an avatar in the inexorable progress of science and medicine. Anchoring will also play an important role in the opposition to vaccination, as we will see below.

Social representations are not, however, a set of ideas to which all members of a society would adhere, but constitute points of reference on which oppositions are organised, "principles generating positions".[5] For example, vaccination can be seen as something effective and good for health (including public health) or as a dangerous attack on bodily integrity. In positioning themselves in this space, people define themselves by assimilation to members of an ingroup, i.e. those who think like them, and by contrast to an outgroup with whom they disagree. For example, in Chapter 3, we saw that seeing vaccination as effective and beneficial to public health could enhance an identity as "reasonable people" as distinct from "anti-vax", "anti-science" figures, who are at the other end of the continuum. For those who are more critical of vaccination, in contrast, the opposition between "science" and "obscurantism" does not apply to their representation of vaccination. Instead, many of them claim to adhere to science and put forward a "critical" vision of science, which would value debate and individual questioning (to which they adhere) over an institutionalised, fixed (and even financially polluted) vision of science. By placing themselves on the 'critical' pole, these individuals also define a *shared point of reference* (critical spirit rather than obscurantism) at the basis of a collective positioning of the group in relation to other actors. We are of course thinking of "official scientists" who would not give up their certainties, or more generally of "sheep" who refuse to look reality in the eyes.

In this perspective, social representations do not characterise consensual opinions or beliefs, but rather "terrains", "issues" on which everyone positions themselves. The social insertion of individuals will play a role in the attachment they give to certain "organising principles" and in their positioning in relation to them. For example, abortion can be seen from the point of view of the principle of respect for life (principle 1) or from the point of view of the woman's freedom (principle 2). A Christian fundamentalist will probably position herself more on the first principle while a feminist student will more readily position herself on the second. As we can see, the study of social representations links sociology to psychology.

According to this approach, the representations of the vaccine and vaccination could not be conceived as a reflection of a lack of knowledge or as the simple result of intra-individual cognitive biases. On the contrary, representations are socially shared within a community and their determinants must therefore be found in the social context. And far from reflecting a lack of knowledge, an impoverished image of its object, they contribute on the contrary to enriching it, by associating particular social meanings to it (as when the vaccine is seen as the materialization of a social relationship).

SOCIAL REPRESENTATIONS OF VACCINATION

Vaccination is a challenge to common sense, as it involves transmitting the virus, or parts of it, to combat its own spread. It is possible to identify certain representations commonly associated with vaccination, although care should be taken as representations vary according to the vaccine under consideration. Moreover, few studies have addressed these issues by explicitly focusing on research into social representations. We will therefore rely mainly on examples from other fields of research. One exception is a research study[6] which examined the social representation of vaccination among pro- and anti-vaccine French people. Respondents were asked to indicate the five words that came most quickly to mind when the word 'vaccine' was mentioned. This collection method is based on an approach to social representations[7] in which a distinction is made between the central "core", i.e. a set of stable, shared and non-negotiable elements, and the "periphery", which are more flexible, dynamic and likely to vary according to the individual. For the pro-vaxxers, the core was characterised by terms such as "disease", "protection", "health". The periphery referred to concepts that interpreted the role of the vaccine in a positive sense: "prevention", "effective", "useful", etc. For the anti-vaxxers (significantly fewer in the study), the central core included the word 'poison'. The periphery shed light on things using terms such as "aluminium", "metals" (in reference to the supposedly dangerous adjuvants used in vaccines), "handicap", "death", "disease", etc. More generally, the representations of the pros focused more on collective issues, the "person" being linked to society as a whole, and trust therefore playing a leading role. On the other hand, among the anti-vaxxers, it was the "fear" of the individual's body being damaged that dominated. Vaccines were seen as a way of bringing about disease and even death. These data thus reveal a conflict between trust/

community *versus* fear/individual, although a larger study would be needed to confirm these results.

DOES EACH VACCINE HAVE ITS OWN SOCIAL REPRESENTATION?

Vaccine hesitancy does not necessarily affect all vaccines. Very different social representations can affect different vaccines. Take the example of Gardasil, the vaccine to prevent cervical cancer, a sexually transmitted disease caused by the human papillomavirus (HPV). This vaccine must be administered before the first sexual intercourse and therefore also to boys. This vaccine questions specific representations regarding the "virginity" of adolescents and, specifically, of young girls. Parents who simply do not consider the possibility of sexual intercourse for their child before the age of 18 see little point in having their child vaccinated before the age of 13, an age at which sexuality has not yet been discussed with their children. Indeed, some studies[8] suggest that one of the main barriers for parents is precisely that HPV vaccination would be perceived as encouraging sexual activity, a conclusion largely contradicted by the evidence.[9] Such barriers are, of course, likely to be more difficult to overcome in communities that cultivate very strict norms regarding the sexuality of young girls. As can be seen, specific issues characterise each vaccine depending on the disease targeted, the age of vaccination, the audience reached, etc.

The fact that social representations vary from one vaccine to another and lead to a form of selectivity in the people who show vaccine hesitancy partly reflects the processes of diffusion of social representations. Social representations are propagated in part through the media. The "traditional" media are often reluctant to relay positions opposed to vaccination. The same is true for movements or personalities with significant political "capital" whose credibility could be damaged by an association with the "anti-vax". Ward and Peretti-Watel[10] note that one strategy adopted by anti-vaccination movements is to target specific vaccines while denying the "anti-vaccination" label. For example, the alleged risk posed by aluminium-containing "adjuvants"[11] has found resonance in the media and with an environmentalist member of the European Parliament. But as we have seen, the same vaccine can also be the subject of divergent representations. Thus, Gardasil can be characterised in very different ways:

> Gardasil can be presented both as a HPV vaccine, an example of how vaccination in general saves millions of lives, one of the few vaccines that contain aluminium, one of the vaccines against sexually transmitted diseases (such as hepatitis B), a recent vaccine or one of the only vaccines recommended for under-18s that is not mandatory.

Each of these characterisations corresponds to distinct anchors that refer to particular norms and attitudes. Thus, a "recent" vaccine would require more "testing", a vaccine containing aluminium would necessarily be dangerous, etc. In short, even if "vaccines" or "vaccination" in general can be the object of social representations, we can identify differentiated representations according to the specific vaccine. In the following section, however, we will consider certain common anchors in relation to vaccination.

VACCINATION, "WAR" AND "GENOCIDE"

In 2003 and 2004, there were smear campaigns against polio vaccination in Nigeria. The rhetoric behind these revolts presented vaccination as 'anti-Islamic' and as a Western move to decimate Muslim populations. It was seen as an extension of the wars in Bosnia and Iraq, with the same alleged objective. In this context, opposition to vaccination is seen as an act of resistance or guerrilla warfare. This image is also used by anti-vaccination movements, which have made extensive use of World War II analogies to characterise public policies for managing the epidemic. Containment decisions were likened to those of fascist regimes, or even to the setting up of "concentration camps" (according to the activist Tal Schaller), with anti-vaxxers claiming to be "resistance fighters". This example illustrates that the representation of the vaccine (seen here as an instrument of surveillance) is part of a more global representation of society.

A related anchor can be identified in certain communities, particularly in or from Africa, which have been the object of large-scale medical experimentation. For some, influenced by this memory, AIDS is a disease introduced by the West to decimate African populations by killing them or rendering them sterile. It may be tempting to incorporate the COVID-19 vaccination into such a narrative. By seeing it as another "large-scale experiment" by the West, it is anchored in an anti-colonial representation.

One of the most widely shared representations of the COVID-19 epidemic has been the suggestion that it aims to impose a "new world order". This borrows a term used by the World Economic Forum (WEF) in Davos but twists it. According to this view, the COVID-19 epidemic is used as a pretext to dismantle the open capitalist economy and create a single government that would control the entire world population. Vaccination is sometimes seen as an adjunct to this goal. In this case, we can see that it is rooted in eugenicist practices such as those practised in the United States at the beginning of the 20th century[12] or later by the Nazis. Thus, Tucker Carlson, the presenter of the influential conservative American channel *Fox News*, suggested on 18 December 2020 that administering the (new) Pfizer vaccine to health professionals was "eugenics" as most were people of very modest origin. In the same vein, a participant in the French study mentioned above wrote: "compulsory vaccination is a strategy to eliminate as many people as possible, without any visible war". The idea that vaccination would contribute to this goal is an extension of this vision.

VACCINATION AND FINANCIAL INTERESTS

A common thread in anti-vaccination discourse is that the vaccine is viewed from a commercial perspective, polluted by conflicts of interest. Vaccines can then be linked to worlds such as "Big Pharma", corruption, profit, etc. In this perspective, political authorities, control agencies and even the WHO would be to varying degrees under the sway of such financial interests, which would dictate their decisions on health matters. Thus, during the H1N1 epidemic, *Pharmacologue X* protested against the French government's vaccination policy in a text shared on many websites[13]: "the strategy is always the same: to instrumentalise the WHO via working groups created, financed, and infiltrated by the pharmaceutical industry." This is despite the fact that the vaccine in question is allegedly dangerous and the pharmacovigilance data is worrying. Of course, this theme was particularly prominent during the COVID-19 pandemic. The idea of the 'new world order' fits this vision. Cases of drugs being marketed despite proven dangers or disastrous clinical trials support this type of discourse. Similarly, examples of the financial and business practices of pharmaceutical companies, often concerned with maximising profits or shareholder margins, can also be used to underpin this kind of discourse.

THE UNNATURAL VACCINE

A third anchor consists of seeing vaccines as part of "technology", seen as artificial and dangerous, in opposition to "nature", seen as beneficial to health. In this representation, nature is fundamentally benevolent, which explains a preference for "natural" medicines. This idea is associated with a view that a "healthy" and "natural" lifestyle provides "natural immunity", making vaccination unnecessary. This lifestyle is thus perceived as a much more effective means of prevention than vaccination, a practice which is also associated with other non-natural practices such as eating frozen food, consuming industrial products, etc.[14] It should be noted that this representation can be anchored in other recommended practices, such as breastfeeding, which is considered preferable to bottle-feeding.

The concept of "healthism" proposed by the American sociologist Robert Crawford[15] sheds light on the popularity of this view of the vaccine as "unnatural" and its consequences for vaccination. Crawford refers to an ideology that sees health as a central means of achieving well-being, and that this is achieved (mainly) through lifestyle adjustments. While people who adhere to this ideology recognise that health problems are caused by things outside the individual (e.g. "junk food", advertising, working conditions), they can be solved by behaving in a "healthy" way – by using personal development practices (such as yoga), eating a balanced and healthy diet, and exercising. The prevalence of this social representation also explains why vaccination is much less popular among practitioners of wellness and self-help techniques as well as among followers of "alternative medicine" (such as naturopathy, homeopathy, etc.).[16]

According to Crawford, by placing a central value on health and neglecting the role of social factors in solving these problems, "healthism" turns out to be a conservative political ideology. For example, obesity, which is more prevalent among certain socio-economically disadvantaged groups, will be seen as a problem that can be solved by "healthy living" and improved dietary practices. It will also fail to question the social inequalities that may partly explain this phenomenon (for example, the cost of access to food, "food deserts", the lack of quality school canteens, poorly calibrated prevention policies, etc.). This healthism is therefore based on a social representation of health that is fundamentally individualistic. On the one hand, the individual is seen as a free and autonomous being, responsible for his or her health choices. This posture therefore conflicts with public health policies that use coercion to achieve vaccination coverage. On the other hand, the idea prevails that each individual is fundamentally different, depending on his or her physiological and anatomical characteristics but also on his or her lifestyle. This approach is therefore at odds with a vaccination policy that would apply to entire segments of a population without consideration for singular characteristics. It also explains the fact that people who are hesitant often rely on their doctor, who is supposed to know them in their "uniqueness", as illustrated by this response from a mother explaining why she did not have her daughter vaccinated: "my daughter was lactose intolerant for the first few years of her life. We did not vaccinate her with MMR because she was very weak." Interestingly, when parents are asked about their reasons for not having their child vaccinated, they often refer to the specific characteristics of their child, or their child's health trajectory,[17] as this example illustrates. These parents are therefore not necessarily opposed to vaccination. They may even be very much in favour of it . . . but not for their child.

VACCINE AND FREEDOM

If there is one theme that has strongly animated campaigns against vaccination, it is that of freedom. As vaccination is a personal choice, it cannot be imposed or subjected to constraints or benefits (such as the *health pass* in France or the *COVID-safe ticket* in Belgium). This valorisation of freedom is not limited to the followers of personal development. It can be found in libertarian and even extreme right-wing movements, which are particularly concerned about the State's hold on individual freedoms. The latter were severely undermined during the COVID-19 pandemic. Vaccine policy can easily be associated with the liberticidal measures taken to curb the pandemic. While criticism of measures to restrict freedoms is perfectly legitimate, it can also be accompanied by conspiracy theories such as the aforementioned "new world order" theory. This emphasis on freedom partly explains the surprising convergence, during the COVID-19 pandemic, between communities devoted to well-being and personal development, which are often not very political (or are close to environmentalist circles), and far-right libertarian movements.

VACCINE AND PROVIDENCE

Among some fundamentalist religious groups, there is an anchor that vaccination should be denounced because it interferes with divine providence. If you are sick, you *must* be sick. To seek to prevent it is to defy God's will. This discourse is sometimes accompanied by a moralising view of vaccines, especially those that prevent STDs. In this case, the disease is seen as a legitimate punishment for the "sin" of the flesh (adultery, homosexuality, etc.) and vaccinating would encourage these practices.

While the concept of divine providence has historically played an important role in anti-vaccination mobilisations, this representation is now limited to very small, often fundamentalist groups. Although lower rates of vaccination are found in some religious communities, studies suggest that this belief does not play a central role. Nevertheless, it is questionable whether the "healthism" already mentioned is not a form of secularisation of these ideas. After all, by giving health a moral value, healthism also suggests that if we are sick, it is because we have behaved in such a way as to be sick. Returning to its etymological roots, health is seen as equivalent to divine salvation.

VACCINES AND THE REPRESENTATION OF SCIENCE

The social representations of vaccination can also be seen in the more general context of those concerning science. Although the concept of science is in fact rather vague, surveys on this topic (in France and Great Britain in particular) show that, for ordinary people, the biomedical sciences play a central role.[18] Medicine is seen as the "science par excellence". It is therefore not surprising that attitudes towards vaccination are closely linked to general views of science. In a recent study,[19] people who gave more credence to science were also those who were most likely to be vaccinated against COVID-19. However, trust in science has declined significantly since the late 1970s. This can be explained by various health crises (contaminated blood, mad cow disease, etc.) or technological crises (Fukushima, etc.) which have shown the limits of science but also cast doubt on the disinterested nature of scientists. Work shows that these crises led to the merging of two previously distinct images of the scientist, namely that of the scientist in the service of the common good (exemplified by Louis Pasteur) and that of the mad scientist· (exemplified by Dr Frankenstein).[20] The links between research laboratories and either states or private companies, as well as the disasters attributed to technology, have undermined this distinction.

When studying representations of science, it is important to distinguish between the scientific process on the one hand and science as an institution on the other (with its locus of power). As we saw in Chapter 3, pro-vaccination people often claim to be scientists. But this is also true of many people who are opposed to vaccination and who claim to adhere to the scientific process. The latter is then seen as a rational, disinterested undertaking, not polluted by financial concerns or power issues. It is therefore science as an institution that is distrusted.[21] The combination of confidence in the scientific process and distrust of the science institution has several consequences. First of all, the "scientific consensus", i.e. the knowledge on which the vast majority of the scientific community agrees in a particular field, may then appear suspicious because it may be influenced by the power dynamics at work in this institution. With the conspiracism that easily infiltrates attitudes towards science, and this is the second consequence, figures who oppose this consensus, far from being seen as cranks, can be valued, seeing their positions given legitimacy. This is the case of Andrew Wakefield, principal author of the fraudulent *Lancet* article on the link between the MMR vaccine and autism, Luc Montagnier, Nobel Prize winner for the discovery of the AIDS virus, and Didier Raoult, both of whom are highly regarded by the anti-vaccination movements. The *leaders* of the anti-vaccination movements are often general practitioners and scientists, whose CVs are sometimes impressive. Such disagreements can be used to show that consensus is illusory. By refusing to listen to "dissonant views", members of the *establishment* would effectively betray the ideals of openness and transparent debate that are supposed to characterise science.

It is tempting to blame negative attitudes towards certain technological innovations on a lack of knowledge. In this "deficit" model, ignorance of the scientific process is blamed for vaccine hesitancy. This view is unsatisfactory. Opponents to vaccination are often very informed on the subject, and, as indicated in Chapter 1, vaccine hesitant people are not necessarily the least educated. Moreover, with regard to the individualised conception of science, "healthism", the question is not only about scientific knowledge, but also about the orientations that guide research. For parents, it is a question of whether there is enough research on children *like their own*. They recognise the benefit-risk ratio in general, but this statistical reality says nothing about the benefit-risk ratio for their child.

Some recent work also suggests that *spirituality* plays a role in resistance to vaccination.[22] In secularised Western societies, fewer and fewer people are active in institutionalised religious groups. Instead, many value "spirituality". In other words, there is a sense that "something is beyond us" without necessarily being part of a religion. Spirituality is characterised by a relationship to the world that suggests that truth cannot be approached solely through reason (and science). Personal and individual experience plays a central role. These beliefs are also widely shared among followers of personal development, already mentioned. Unsurprisingly, there is a positive relationship between scepticism about vaccination and defining oneself as a spiritually attached person.

VACCINE RUMOURS

"Tetanus vaccine makes you sterile". Why did this rumour circulate from 1994 onwards, contributing to a significant reduction in vaccination coverage in several Catholic countries? Because a member of an anti-IVG Catholic movement and "provie" had misinterpreted a scientific article reporting a contraceptive vaccine using a protein also used in the tetanus vaccine. His interpretation, rather than the actual result of the article, spread to the public, raising fears about the vaccine. At the time of writing, many young people in Britain, France, Belgium claim to have been stung in nightclubs and to have experienced various symptoms subsequently.[23] While many victims have come forward, no evidence of such practices or arrest of suspects has been reported to date. It is therefore difficult to know whether these rumours are true.

The concept of rumour refers to "a statement intended to be believed, relating to current events and spread without official verification".[24] The notion of rumour emphasises the dissemination of information within a network of individuals, often by word of mouth. While this aspect of dissemination is characteristic of rumours, they can nevertheless be considered as social representations. Each vaccine rumour is part of a representation of the world and a form of appropriation of "science" by common sense.

One of the characteristics of rumours is their tendency to change as they are disseminated, often to match widely shared representations. For example, in a famous experiment,[25] white American participants were shown an image of a scene in an underground train. Among the passengers, all seated, a well-dressed black man was talking with a white man holding a razor. The subjects were asked to describe the scene to another subject, using the "Arab phone" principle. The evolution of these descriptions was carefully analysed. And what was the result? After a few steps, the roles were reversed in half of the "chains": the white man was described as well dressed and the black man was holding the razor. In other words, according to a principle described by the English psychologist Bartlett as "conventionalization", the rumour gradually came to conform to common beliefs and representations. Stereotypes, i.e. beliefs about the traits possessed by a social group, play an important role in this respect. They dictate expectations about the target group[26] and can lead to our perception of a scene or story being transformed in the direction of these expectations.

If rumours are passed on, some are even transposed from one context to another. For example, the idea that one vaccine is being used to sterilise the population may be recycled in relation to another vaccine. In Kenya, for example, the tetanus vaccine was blamed in the 1990s and the polio vaccine was blamed in 2015.[27] Similarly, the idea that consuming bleach (a very bad idea!) helps combat autism supposedly triggered by the MMR (measles-mumps-rubella) vaccine has been recycled in the context of COVID-19 (and even relayed by Donald Trump).

One of the most famous rumours in the field of vaccination is that of a link between the MMR vaccine and autism. This myth, which dates back to the early 1990s, was given scientific backing through the work of British researcher Andrew Wakefield, author of a study "proving" the link and published in one of the most prestigious medical journals, *The Lancet*, in 1998. This publication had a devastating effect on vaccination coverage in several countries. The digital revolution has helped spread the rumour to every corner of the world. Yet the study was fraudulent and tainted by conflicts of interest, leading the journal to withdraw the article in 2005. Subsequent studies have confirmed that there is no link between MMR vaccination and autism.

The popularity of this rumour can be explained by well-known psychological processes. On the one hand, MMR vaccination coincides with the age at which the first signs of autism are identified. When two phenomena follow each other and a causal explanation is available to account for this succession, it is obviously tempting to invoke it. If on the day you first put on your new hairstyle, the person who makes your pulse race compliments you on your appearance, will you not tend to see your expensive trip to your eminent hairdresser as responsible for this praise? This is the famous *post hoc ergo propter hoc* bias we have already seen in Chapter 2. But the explanation is not only cognitive. From an emotional point of view, a diagnosis of autism is a blow to which families look for an explanation. Blaming vaccination makes it possible to identify an external and controllable cause and to identify those responsible (the pharmaceutical lobby in particular) who are "pulling the strings". This rumour is accompanied by a conspiracy theory, as is often the case. The popularity of the rumour is based on collective dynamics. For example, Wakefield was particularly influential in communities of Somali origin (especially in the state of Minnesota), where there was a high rate of autism. Studies of these communities have shown that mothers shared their fears about the vaccine.[28] Note that rumours are not necessarily false. Sometimes true information is spread through rumours before it is validated by the authorities. For example, the WHO's monitoring of smallpox was based on a "rumour register".[29] And for good reason! One case would have been enough to call into question the eradication of the disease. It was therefore necessary to be quick on the ball and to capitalise on rumours to react. Similarly, in 2004, cases of avian flu were detected thanks to rumours, allowing to prevent a larger epidemic.

In contexts where information is locked up and/or the information offered by "official" channels is unreliable, rumours naturally gain in importance. According to two American social psychologists, Allport and Postman, the fundamental law of rumour is that the intensity and spread of a rumour depends on its importance multiplied by the ambiguity of the available evidence. Importance is based on a subjective feeling and has a central emotional dimension. As for evidence, the more inconclusive or contradictory the evidence on the efficacy or safety of a vaccine, the easier it is for a rumour to take hold. Obviously, access to masses of information, especially online, only accentuates this feeling.

In light of this law, rumours are especially likely to emerge when new vaccines are used and, in particular, when they use novel technologies such as messenger RNA. For example, rumours that Pfizer and Moderna vaccines transform the DNA of their hosts may have fuelled fears about them and discouraged many people from getting vaccinated. Rumours are more likely to spread the more socially significant their subject matter, as was the case during the COVID-19 pandemic.[30]

CONSPIRACY THEORIES AND VACCINATION

In 2021, in France, the Servier laboratories were condemned in the Mediator scandal, an anti-diabetic drug responsible for the deaths of more than 1,000 people. Several executives of the company continued to market the drug despite the danger and the drug safety regulator was negligent, to say the least. We are thus faced with a collusion of actors determined to harm others in order to enrich the company's accounts (and themselves), in short, a conspiracy. Conspiracies in the medical-pharmaceutical world can be identified in a few instances. Despite the safeguards, the financial stakes, sometimes enormous, can incite certain malicious people to collude to the detriment of the public's health. But if conspiracies exist, it is important to distinguish them from a vastly more common phenomenon of a psychosocial nature, that of conspiracy theories. A conspiracy theory is a belief, whereas a conspiracy is a fact.

A conspiracy theory can be defined as "a claim that the public is intentionally misled about some aspect of reality in order to enable a group to secretly implement an ill-intentioned and self-serving agenda".[31] For example, the belief that vaccination is used to implant computer chips to monitor the population is a conspiracy theory because it assumes that the experts (who claim that vaccination is beneficial) are knowingly lying in order to allow pharmaceutical and technology firms to enrich themselves. The conspiracy theory thus implies on the one hand a hidden conspiracy, but also a deliberate undertaking to conceal reality on the part of agents who collaborate in the conspiracy, or even benefit from it.

As with rumours, conspiracy theories about vaccination can be seen as part of social representations. These shared representations are indeed a form of appropriation of science by common sense. Conspiracy theories often target groups that are considered powerful. As in populist discourse, they are often based on a segmentation of society between the "elites" and the "people". On the one hand, there are political leaders, the "mainstream" media, big business leaders, academics and recognised experts, etc. Although diverse, these agents would be linked to each other. The media and scientists would collaborate to conceal plots secretly hatched by financiers and politicians. In this view, the elites are necessarily treacherous and concerned only with their own self-interest. Conversely, the people would be benevolent but naive. They would be content to follow the path laid out by the elites without realising that this is contrary to their own interests. Hence the metaphor of the "sheep". From this group, a small category of "enlightened" individuals, the conspiracy theorists, stand out, who have allegedly cracked the mystery and uncovered the plot.[32] Conspiracy theory is a syndrome in that people who subscribe to one conspiracy theory often tend to subscribe to others. Indeed, each conspiracy theory offers elements that support other conspiracy theories. For example, if the US government organised the 9/11 conspiracies to justify an invasion of Iraq for the benefit of the military-industrial complex, this same power probably also seeks to enrich itself on the backs of its citizens through bribes offered by pharmaceutical firms to those who would organise vaccination campaigns at great expense. This explains the popularity of anti-vaccination conspiracy theories that feed on other already popular theories. It may also explain why belief in conspiracy theories that are totally unrelated to vaccination (e.g., the death of Lady Di) show a consistent association with vaccine hesitancy across many countries.[33]

Vaccination campaigns are particularly fertile ground for the emergence of conspiracy theories. These campaigns are necessarily organised by political authorities, often far away, and involve pharmaceutical companies. Moreover, despite the considerable resources deployed to carry out these campaigns, the direct benefits of vaccination are not always immediately apparent, raising suspicions about the motives of the individuals orchestrating them. The less trust one has in the authorities, the more likely one is to subscribe to conspiracy theories by implicating the authorities.[34] Conversely, the spread of conspiracy theories undermines trust in the authorities and in those associated with "evil elites". In 2003–2004, there was a boycott of the polio vaccination campaign in northern Nigeria. The boycott, initiated by the governors of three states, lasted eleven months. The boycott was not because of any specific problems with the polio vaccine, but because of what the vaccine represented. The Nigerian government was seen to be complicit with powerful Western authorities, who were widely distrusted. According to one local doctor, the vaccine had been "corrupted and tainted by American evildoers and their Western allies".[35] In general, many anti-vaccination movements show a lack of trust in the authorities, and sometimes for very legitimate reasons!

It should be noted that the capital of trust (or distrust) of people adhering to conspiracy theories is not distributed equally to all the actors involved in vaccination. A study conducted in Belgium at the beginning of the COVID-19 pandemic revealed that people characterised by a "conspiracy mentality" harboured a particularly marked distrust of political authorities and scientific experts.[36] In contrast, no link emerged between conspiracism and distrust of medical personnel. In direct contact with their patients, the latter come across as less likely to be under the sway of financial or political interests. In fact, the study also suggests that the relationship between conspiracy and distrust of scientists and authorities is based on the perception that the latter *are using the pandemic* for their own benefit, which is less the case for medical personnel.

IS THE POWER OF CONSPIRACY THEORIES IN SHAPING ANTI-VACCINE ATTITUDES OVERESTIMATED?

We have suggested so far that endorsement of a conspiracist world-view may incline people to distrust vaccines and, hence, fail to vaccinate. While this is perfectly plausible, most of the studies on this topic have relied on cross-sectional studies, i.e., measuring conspiracy beliefs and vaccination intentions (or vaccination status) at the same time. This means that it is difficult to establish a causal relationship between both variables (correlation does not mean causation!). Actually, the reverse proposition, that vaccine hesitancy would facilitate endorsement of conspiracy theories is not without merits. As we have seen, people may have many motives for failing to vaccinate: some of these have nothing to do with conspiracy theories. For example, having been afraid of syringes since one's early childhood. While such people may be initially reluctant to vaccinate due to such fears, they may come to justify or rationalize such fears by adhering to conspiracy theories. These may seem more "rational" or socially acceptable than admitting their fear of syringes for example. To address this possibility, it is important to evaluate vaccination intentions and conspiracy beliefs at multiple time points. This is exactly what van Prooijen and Böhm[37] have done in both the Netherlands and the US during the COVID-19 pandemic. In the Netherlands, they find evidence for both mechanisms: conspiracy beliefs at time 1 did predict later Vaccination intentions but the reverse was true as well. In the US, they only found support for the "rationalization" hypothesis: vaccination intentions predicted later adhesion to conspiracy beliefs but not vice versa. Obviously, this has implications for interventions against vaccine hesitancy: conspiracy beliefs may sometimes be a symptom or manifestation of vaccine hesitancy rather than its root.

Another line of work qualifying the role of conspiracy theories in shaping vaccination behaviour comes from work conducted by

German researchers.[38] Across several studies, these authors showed that the link between conspiracy and the intention to vaccinate was cancelled out if subjective norms were taken into account. In other words, if you believe that those around you think it's important to get vaccinated, you'll get vaccinated a lot more, whatever the level of conspiracism. Conspiracism only predicts people's intention to be vaccinated if they do not perceive any pro-vaccination norms in their environment.

EXPLAINING ADHERENCE TO ANTI-VACCINE THINKING

We have reviewed the three forms of social thinking: social representations, rumours, and conspiracy theories. As you will have noticed, these are not watertight. Social representations serve as ferment for rumours, which can feed conspiracy theories and so on. If we treated them separately, it is above all because the literature on these subjects is rather segmented. The proximity of these three categories invites us to consider the motivations that encourage adherence to these forms of social thought, particularly when they encourage vaccine hesitation. Three main types of motivation can be distinguished.[39]

The first type concerns "epistemic" motivations, i.e. those that lead to an understanding of reality. Conspiracy theories, like social representations in general (through the processes of anchoring and objectification), offer a simple reading of a complex reality. This explains why they are so popular in times of crisis or when dealing with multifactorial social events such as a pandemic. Disease and its consequences are obviously a source of uncertainty. But scientific discoveries that are still little known to the general public (such as RNA vaccines . . .) that aim to respond to them can also fuel these feelings. The same applies to the authorities' procrastination or changes of direction. Work[40] shows that the communication of rumours also fulfils such an epistemic function. These authors analysed Internet chat rooms and found that the exchanges serve to make collective sense of the phenomenon targeted by the rumour. Moreover, conspiracy theories have attractive qualities from an epistemic point of view: they are irrefutable. Indeed, any attempt to challenge them is seen as an attempt to conceal the truth. For example, the fact that so few cases of serious adverse reactions to the COVID-19 vaccines have been identified could be seen as evidence that they have been deliberately hidden, and thus an argument for the harmfulness of vaccines.

The second type concerns "existential" motivations and relates to the need for security and control over one's environment. By understanding an unknown event, one can better control it and feel more secure. Thus, rumours are mostly communicated in situations of anxiety and the process of collective interpretation already mentioned could partly channel this anxiety.[41] Similarly, by unmasking the evil agents that influence our destiny, conspiracy theory could partly neutralise them or reduce the threat they pose. Unfortunately, there is a gap between hope and reality. Studies show that engaging in conspiracism can increase these feelings of anxiety and loss of control.[42] Conspiracism makes the world even more anxiety-provoking, because the reality it describes is itself evanescent. Indeed, behind every conspiracy there may be an even more evil plot. Moreover, plots feed off each other. For a plot by one group to be credible, it is often necessary to invoke the complicity of another group and so on, expanding the list of potential enemies and making the world even more threatening.

The social representations, rumours and conspiracy theories that emerge in times of crisis are often associated with uncertainties. In the case of COVID-19, one thinks of all the worries, even anxieties, that the disease, RNA vaccines or even the procrastination of the authorities may arouse. But such representations can be grafted onto pre-existing concerns unrelated to the pandemic. For example, one technology that is causing concern is the development of 5G, accused by some of transmitting diseases (brain cancer) or being used to "control minds". The observation by a Belgian engineer that the construction of a 5G tower in Wuhan coincided with the start of the epidemic gave rise to the rumour that 5G was responsible for the pandemic (we see the *post ergo propter post hoc* heuristic at work). This was accompanied by the idea that, under the leadership of Bill Gates, the vaccine would be used to implant chips linked to the 5G network and enable population control. The grip of this rumour can be likened to the anchoring process mentioned earlier. This rumour is all the more effective because it is grafted onto existing representations of the dangers of "waves".

A third type of motivation is also social in that it is about building social relationships and maintaining a good image of oneself and one's community. Spreading rumours or conspiracy theories can help to integrate socially if the rumours are interesting or reinforce views already valued in the group.[43] Spreading a rumour about the dangers of vaccination can give the feeling that one is offering valuable information to one's audience in order to preserve one's own health or that of one's relatives. In short, one confirms one's status within the group. In the same spirit, conspiracy theories have a very valuable characteristic: they are entertaining. In one study,[44] the procedure involved reading an account of the death of billionaire paedophile Jeffrey Epstein. The text was manipulated to make it appear that he was the victim of a conspiracy or that he committed suicide. The account was considered more entertaining in the first condition. Despite the macabre content of the text, the feedback even reported more positive emotional experiences when a plot was mentioned. As mentioned above, being a conspiracist (even if this term is rejected by the people it refers to!) allows one to feel valued and to be part of an 'elite' of "enlightened" people, distinguishing oneself from "sheep".

In general, social representations, rumours and conspiracy theories serve a function of social differentiation (see Chapter 3), as they portray the ingroup in a positive light in comparison to other groups, which will be readily denigrated. Think of conspiracy theories about "Big Pharma" being venal and opposed to "good people who crave freedom", or the idea that the conspiracy is a weapon of the Chinese government (opposing here Westerners who love democracy and freedom). Rumours about COVID-19 and vaccination often make use of stereotypes and prejudices that devalue 'outgroups', thus highlighting our own community. As is often the case, antisemitism has taken pride of place. Historically, Jews were seen as responsible for the transmission of the plague in the 14th century or cholera in the 19th century.[45] Today, antisemitism takes different forms. Anti-vaccination activists (especially in Germany) have been seen wearing Stars of David. In this way, one presents oneself as a victim of a "holocaust", usurping in the process their victim status from Jews during the Second World War. Antisemitism can also manifest itself in the idea of a global "grand conspiracy". The "new world order" conspiracy theory is an example of this. It borrows a term used by the World Economic Forum (WEF) in Davos, but misuses it. According to this theory, the COVID-19 epidemic is used as a pretext to dismantle the open capitalist economy and create a single government that would control the entire world population. This theory is similar to the idea of the "global Jewish conspiracy", a classic conspiracy theory, and gives pride of place to figures from the world of finance, a universe linked to Jewishness in representations. Moreover, the WEF is often perceived in these discourses as "controlled by Jews".[46]

The COVID-19 pandemic has undoubtedly contributed to such social motivations by destructuring the social environment of many of us, through confinement and teleworking, and even by excluding certain people (unvaccinated, sick people, contact cases, people who have lost their jobs or who have been forced to telework . . .) from many spheres of public life. Basically, under the cover of this pandemic, many individuals have discovered new communities of belonging and places of socialisation. These social motivations certainly explain why stigmatising those who are on the "fringe", who "doubt" (people who are reluctant to be vaccinated against COVID-19 without being radically anti-vax), is likely to reinforce adherence to movements of a conspiracy nature. The latter offer a potentially rewarding response to these social motivations. However, it must be admitted that such benefits are probably less palpable through adherence to the "official discourse".

NOTES

1 Rouquette, M.-L. (2009). Introduction: Qu'est-ce que la pensée sociale? [Introduction: What is social thought?]. In Rouquette, M.-L. (Dir.), *La Pensée sociale*. Toulouse, France: Eres.

2 Moscovici, S. (2008). *Psychoanalysis: Its image, its public*. New York: Polity Press.

3 Tavani, J. L., Piermattéo, A., Monaco, G. L., & Delouvée, S. (2021). Skepticism and defiance: Assessing credibility and representations of science. *PLOS One*, 16(9).

4 www.newyorker.com/news/q-and-a/when-parents-forbid-the-covid-vaccine.

5 Doise, W., Clémence, A., & Lorenzi-Cioldi, F. (1992). *Représentations sociales et analyse de données* [Social representations and data analysis]. Grenoble: Presses universitaires de Grenoble.

6 Gaymard, S., & Hidrio, R. (2020). Sphères publiques et représentations sociales du vaccin. Analyse chez les pro-vaccins et les anti-vaccins [Public spheres and social representations of the vaccine]. *Communication: Information Media Practical Theory*, 37(2).

7 Flament, C. (1989). Structure et Dynamique des representations sociales [Structure and dynamics of social representations]. In *Les Représentations sociales*. Paris: Presses universitaires de France.

8 Ezeanochie, M. C., & Olagbuji, B. N. (2014). Human papilloma virus vaccine: Determinants of acceptability by mothers for adolescents in Nigeria. *African Journal of Reproductive Health*, 18(3), 154–158.

9 Brewer, N. T., Hall, M. E., Malo, T. L., Gilkey, M. B., Quinn, B., & Lathren, C. (2017). Announcements versus conversations to improve HPV vaccination coverage: A randomized trial. *Pediatrics*, 139(1).

10 Ward, J. K., & Peretti-Watel, P. (2020). Comprendre la méfiance vis-à-vis des vaccins: Des biais de perception aux controverses [Understanding vaccine distrust: From perception bias to controversy]. *Revue Française de Sociologie*, 61(2), 243–273.

11 This fear is not justified. WHO considers that there is no reason to question the safety of the many vaccines containing aluminium.

12 Gould, S. J. (1996). *The Mis-measure of Man*. New York: Norton.

13 Ward, J. K. (2017). Vaccine criticism at the time of the A(H1N1) vaccine: Comparing comparisons. *Social Science and Health*, 35(4), 37–59.

14 Attwell, K., Smith, D. T., & Ward, P. R. (2018). 'The unhealthy other': How vaccine-rejecting parents construct the vaccinating mainstream. *Vaccine*, 36(12), 1621–1626.

15 Crawford, R. (1980). Healthism and the medicalization of everyday life. *International Journal of Health Services*, 10(3), 365388.

16 *Ibid*.

17 Goldenberg, M. J. (2016). Public misunderstanding of science? Reframing the problem of vaccine hesitancy. *Perspectives on Science*, 24(5), 552–581.

18 Durant, J., Evans, G., & Thomas, G. (1992). Public understanding of science in Britain: The role of medicine in the popular representation of science. *Public Understanding of Science*, 1(2), 161–182.

19 Tavani, J. L. *et al.* (2021). *Op. cit.*

20 Boy, D. (2014). Les réprésentations sociales de la science [The social representations of science]. In Wievorka, M. (Ed.), *La Science en question(s)* [Science in questions] (pp. 165–183). Paris: Editions Sciences Humaines.

21 Goldenberg, M. J. (2016). *Op. cit.*

22 Rutjens, B. T., Sengupta, N., Der Lee, R. V., van Koningsbruggen, G. M., Martens, J. P., Rabelo, A., & Sutton, R. M. (2022). Science skepticism across 24 countries. *Social Psychological and Personality Science*, 13(1), 102–117.

23 www.lesoir.be/444440/article/2022-05-24/le-phenomene-des-piqures-sauvages-entre-psychose-et-enquetes#:~:text=Souvent%20évoqué%20sur%20les%20réseaux,définir%20l%27éventuelle%20substance%20injectée.

24 Knapp as cited in Delouvée, S. (2018). *Manuel visual de psychologie sociale* [Visual handbook of social psychology]. Paris: Dunod, p. 135.

25 Allport, G. W., & Postman, L. (1947). *The psychology of rumor*. New York: Henry Holt.

26 Yzerbyt, V., & Demoulin, S. (2019). *Les relations intergroupes* [Intergroup relations]. Grenoble: Presses universitaires de Grenoble.

27 Larson, H. J. (2020). *Stuck: How vaccine rumors start and why they don't go away*. Oxford, UK: Oxford University Press.

28 *Ibid.*

29 *Ibid.*

30 Pertwee, E., Simas, C., & Larson, H. J. (2022). An epidemic of uncertainty: Rumors, conspiracy theories and vaccine hesitancy. *Nature Medicine*, 28(3), 456–459.

31 Nera, K., & Schöpfer, C. (2023). What is so special about conspiracy theories? Conceptually distinguishing beliefs in conspiracy theories from conspiracy beliefs in psychological research. *Theory & Psychology*, 33(3), 287–305.

32 Franks, B., Bangerter, A., Bauer, M. W., Hall, M., & Noort, M. C. (2017). Beyond 'monologicality'? Exploring conspiracist worldviews. *Frontiers in Psychology*, 8, 861.

33 Hornsey, M. J., Harris, E. A., & Fielding, K. S. (2018). The psychological roots of anti-vaccination attitudes: A 24-nation investigation. *Health Psychology*, 37(4), 307–315. https://doi.org/10.1037/hea0000586.

34 Van Oost, P., Yzerbyt, V., Schmitz, M., Vansteenkiste, M., Luminet, O., Morbée, S., Van den Bergh, O., Waterschoot, J., & Klein, O. (2022). The relation

between conspiracism, government trust, and COVID-19 vaccination intentions: The key role of motivation. *Social Science & Medicine*, 301, 114926.

35 Jegede, A. S. (2007). What led to the Nigerian boycott of the polio vaccination campaign? *PLOS Medicine*, 4(3).

36 Nera, K., Mora, Y. L., Klein, P., Roblain, A., Van Oost, P., Terache, J., & Klein, O. (2022). Looking for ties with secret agendas during the pandemic: Conspiracy mentality is associated with reduced trust in political, medical, and scientific institutions-but not in medical personnel. *Psychologica Belgica*, 62(1), 193–207.

37 van Prooijen, J. W., & Böhm, N. (in press). Do conspiracy theories shape or rationalize vaccination hesitancy over time? *Social Psychological and Personality Science*. https://doi.org/10.1177/19485506231181659.

38 Winter, K., Pummerer, L., Hornsey, M. J., & Sassenberg, K. (2022). Provaccination subjective norms moderate the relationship between conspiracy mentality and vaccination intentions. *British Journal of Health Psychology*, 27(2), 390–405.

39 Douglas, K. M., Sutton, R. M., & Cichocka, A. (2017). The psychology of conspiracy theories. *Current Directions in Psychological Science*, 26(6), 538–542.

40 Bordia, P., & Difonzo, N. (2004). Problem solving in social interactions on the internet: Rumor as social cognition. *Social Psychology Quarterly*, 67(1), 33–49.

41 Difonzo, N., & Bordia, P. (2007). *Rumor psychology: Social and organizational approaches*. Washington: American Psychological Association.

42 Liekefett, L., Christ, O., & Becker, J. C. (2023). Can conspiracy beliefs be beneficial? Longitudinal linkages between conspiracy beliefs, anxiety, uncertainty aversion, and existential threat. *Personality & Social Psychology Bulletin*, 49(2), 167–179.

43 Difonzo, N., & Bordia, P. (2007). Op. cit.

44 Van Prooijen, J.-W., Ligthart, J., Rosema, S., & Xu, Y. (2022). The entertainment value of conspiracy theories. *British Journal of Psychology*, 113(1), 25–48.

45 Bonhomme, E. (2 May 2021). Germany's anti-vaccination history is riddled with anti-semitism. *The Atlantic*.

46 Anti-Defamation League. (2020). *'The great reset' conspiracy flourishes amid continued pandemic*. www.adl.org/resources/blog/great-reset-conspiracy-flourishes-amid-continued-pandemic.

5

COMBATING VACCINE HESITANCY

On 4 January 2022, two years after the start of the COVID-19 pandemic, French President Emmanuel Macron declared in an interview with *Le Parisien* that he was "very keen to piss off the non-vaccinated" (*sic*). Here is one idea among others to fight against vaccine hesitancy! In Israel, for example, vaccinated young people have been given a drink outside bars, or wireless headphones in Washington. In Quebec, access to liquor and cannabis shops was forbidden if you had not been vaccinated. An inventory of proposals made by vaccination specialists[1] lists 46 items! In this chapter, we will look at possible strategies to address vaccine hesitancy.

Before elaborating on some of these – as a comprehensive review is beyond the scope of this book – a few precautions are necessary. First, we have already discussed the superiority of interventions based on randomised controlled trials (RCTs) over correlational studies in assessing whether or not an intervention is effective (see Box 3.1). Still on the methodological side, another difficulty concerns the purpose of the intervention itself. For ethical and logistical reasons, it is often difficult to conduct a study in which the act of getting vaccinated (the behaviour) is measured. Therefore, we often fall back on the intention to vaccinate. However, as discussed in Chapter 2, while intentions are powerful predictors of subsequent behaviour, moving from words to action is not always straightforward.

Second, on what basis should the effectiveness of an intervention be judged? To say, as in the scientific literature, that the observed result "cannot be explained by chance" is insufficient. Imagine a very expensive advertising campaign to increase HPV vaccination among adolescents that succeeds in increasing the vaccination rate by 0.5%. Even if this result cannot be attributed to chance, it is still disappointing. Clearly, it is not only the *presence of* an intervention's effect that counts, but also its *magnitude*. Unfortunately, interventions are not always as effective as hoped.[2] Why is this? Each potential target of these interventions is constantly faced with a set of constraints that limit behavioural change. Imagine, for example, that you want to convince a smoker to limit his or her tobacco consumption. This will involve fighting against firmly rooted habits (e.g. smoking at lunchtime), which themselves respond to psychological needs (e.g. the stress of a morning's work), and which depend on a particular life situation (e.g. a job requiring constant attention). Faced with the inertia, the "rails" on which such constraints place us, the margin available for psychological intervention to deviate the individual from his or her trajectory is often small. It is therefore all the more important to characterise interventions according to the extent of their effects.

Third, studies evaluating the effectiveness of vaccination campaigns are by definition confined to a particular cultural, historical and social horizon and focus on a specific vaccine and disease. While humans differ somewhat in their responses to a pathogen such as a virus, the diversity of their responses to psychological interventions is immeasurably greater. For example, a video message in English about the dangers of measles from a white American doctor claiming to be from the WHO is likely to be received very differently by a Nigerian farm girl, a German executive and a French shop assistant from Martinique, even though all of them speak Shakespeare's language to some extent. Can we learn from interventions on some people to develop campaigns on others? This question is particularly sensitive because most psychology research has focused on a very small population of rich, educated, industrialised, white people, etc.

All of this explains why, before designing an intervention, it is crucial to work with the target communities. It is important to develop approaches that address their concerns and are consistent with their social and cultural frameworks. The "Majigi" campaign developed in Nigeria in one of the communities where resistance to polio vaccination was highest[3] illustrates this type of approach. It was based on a dialogue with members such as political and religious leaders, traditional healers, birth attendants, town criers and traditional surgeons. The entire community was invited to a community event that began with a prayer, a welcome speech by the village chief, a presentation by the team leader and a play about the consequences of polio. Participants were also shown a PowerPoint presentation and computer simulation on polio transmission, signs, symptoms and complications. Afterwards, participants watched a variety of films that addressed misconceptions about the cause of polio and other negative attitudes towards vaccination. Moving films of polio victims and their relatives showed their frustrations, experiences and disabilities. This was followed by a discussion with the community. The term "Majigi" refers in Hausa (the local language) to film shows conducted by mobile vans, a delivery model familiar to the target community and on which the intervention was based. This integrated approach resulted in a dramatic 310% increase in the percentage of children vaccinated in this community. Clearly, such an intervention was only possible through the involvement of locals within the community and is not transferable as such to other cultural contexts.

As we shall see, in the ocean of literature on vaccine hesitancy, the work that satisfies the three conditions mentioned is, in the end, only a few drops of water. Let us now consider different types of interventions. These can be grouped into four categories. Some interventions focus on beliefs, perceptions and attitudes. A second approach is to increase motivation to vaccinate more directly (e.g. by offering incentives). A third category of interventions aims to act on social processes, relying in particular on social norms (prescriptive or descriptive). Finally, a fourth category of interventions aims to change behaviour directly without going through the motivation to vaccinate.

ACTING ON WHAT PEOPLE THINK

Among the interventions aimed at changing the beliefs and attitudes of individuals who wish to be vaccinated, we will first consider approaches to changing perceptions of the risks associated with the disease (and with vaccination itself). We will then look at interventions targeting vaccine confidence.

ACTING ON RISK PERCEPTION AND FEAR

As discussed in Chapter 2, many people do not get vaccinated because they underestimate the risks associated with the disease, both in terms of the likelihood of becoming infected and the severity of the disease. In February 2020, for example, the Belgian Minister of Health called a virologist warning of the dangers of COVID-19 a "*drama queen*". A logical strategy would therefore be to try to influence this perception of risk in the hope of motivating hesitant people. Unfortunately, attempts to do so have proven unsuccessful.[4]

An impressive study (ECR) of almost 600 German women over 60[5] looked at an important but little-known risk of influenza: sepsis (a serious and potentially fatal infection). Participants were divided into three experimental conditions. In a control condition, there was no intervention. In a second condition, participants had to read a brochure promoting the benefits of vaccination for the elderly. In a third condition, the leaflet was of the same type, but also pointed out the risks of sepsis associated with the flu virus. And, indeed, the result was that the risks of sepsis were more widely known and intentions were altered by reading the leaflet. However, this was not enough to change behaviour. In other words, knowing something is not enough to act, one must be able to implement the behaviour when the opportunity arises and/or actively seek out that opportunity, which is far from obvious. Obstacles are likely to arise at each of these stages, preventing the positive effect on knowledge from materialising.

Beyond changing the perception of risk, a more radical approach is to seek to instil fear. This is the strategy adopted by the authorities when they force cigarette companies to put pictures of smoking-ravaged lungs on cigarette packs. Psychological research shows that, overall, fear appeals can be effective as long as people feel they can act in a meaningful way to deal with the threat. However, there is no research to support this hypothesis in the area of vaccination. Unfortunately, fear appeals can sometimes be counterproductive. First, individuals may seek to avoid the fear – an unpleasant feeling – more than the threat itself, especially if the fear proves difficult to control or avoid. A range of rationalisations or avoidance strategies will emerge – for example, denial of the danger of the virus or a form of fatalism ('there is nothing we can do about it'). Secondly, anxiety-provoking messages can provoke reactions other than fear, and in particular a phenomenon of *reactance*. In fact, during the COVID-19 epidemic, many negative reactions to the "anxiety-provoking" climate created by the media emerged. The fear thus aroused is experienced as an infringement of freedom that can generate anger against the sender of the message and/or the authorities. It is known that such anger has a negative effect on the intention to vaccinate.[6] In sum, there is little evidence to support the idea that appeals to fear promote vaccination among hesitant individuals.

ACTING ON TRUST

Does information about the effectiveness of a vaccine or, conversely, the absence of serious adverse events motivate people to get vaccinated? One of our studies sought to answer this question in January 2021, during the COVID-19 pandemic in Belgium.[7] More than 15,000 internet users were asked to imagine themselves participating in a COVID-19 vaccination campaign. They were asked about their intention to be vaccinated in a situation that varied according to several parameters. These included aspects related to trust. These included efficacy (depending on the condition, the vaccine offered 95% or 70% protection against COVID-19), adverse effects of the vaccine (depending on the condition, no effect, low chance of serious side effects, uncertainty about adverse effects), the place where the vaccination was carried out (at home or in hospital), the probability of transmitting the virus after vaccination, the number of doses (one or two) and social norms (75% vs. 0% of the population already vaccinated). Not surprisingly, vaccination intentions differed significantly according to the scenario presented. But the factors that played the biggest role were efficacy and adverse events. In particular, when there was uncertainty about adverse events, intentions dropped significantly. It should be noted, however, that given the design of this study, it is difficult to know whether the absence of adverse events encouraged hesitancy or whether uncertainty about adverse events discouraged people who would have been willing to be vaccinated. Furthermore, in line with what was mentioned above, this study only assessed vaccination intentions and not behaviour.

While several studies show that various interventions, including educational ones, increase confidence in the vaccine and even vaccine intention, there is little evidence of a robust effect on vaccination itself, especially if one focuses only on studies that use an RCT. Once again, changing beliefs and attitudes is easier than changing behaviour.

RESPONDING TO MISINFORMATION

There has been a lot of false or unsubstantiated information circulated about vaccines, known as "misinformation" or "disinformation". How can this be tackled? There are various interventions that specifically target misinformation about vaccines. These interventions are of two kinds. First, some operate before the misinformation is even exposed. As with vaccination, these approaches aim to prepare people to deal with misinformation by exposing them proactively to examples of misinformation and the reasons why these are false.[8] For example, in March 2021, in the context of the

COVID-19 pandemic, research[9] examined the (unfounded) narrative that messenger RNA vaccines would transform genetic material. This is a fake news that has been widely circulated. The experimental scenario was to present this type of fake news to a group of Canadians over the age of 50. A second group ("inoculation") was informed that some people were spreading such speech, about the strategies used (attacking the authorities, selectively choosing the information that suits them, etc.) and about the reasons why this speech was false. Finally, a control group received no information about vaccination. Vaccination intention was measured before and after the intervention. Unsurprisingly, people who received misinformation were less likely to want to be vaccinated than those in the control group. This was also the case, but to a much lesser extent, in the group exposed to a prior "correction" of misinformation. Early correction of misinformation thus acted as a "vaccine" against the effects of later misinformation.

A second approach is to correct false information after the fact. This is the technique of "fact checking". This approach was used in a study conducted in the United States, Canada and Great Britain, which did not focus specifically on vaccination but on various beliefs related to COVID-19.[10] In the first stage, the subjects' beliefs about various misinformation about the COVID-19 pandemic were collected. The level of agreement was quite high, suggesting that participants had already encountered this information. One group then read a text correcting this information and showing why it was unfounded. Another group saw information that had no relevance to the coronavirus. Unsurprisingly, people in the fact-checking group (but not in the control group) were less likely to buy into the false information after exposure. More remarkably, however, this effect disappeared three months later. Another study compared the effect of an intervention to discredit a conspiracy theory related to vaccination *before* and *after* exposure to it. It showed that belief in the conspiracy theory decreased more when it was preventively discredited.

While some interventions are encouraging, those aimed at correcting misinformation are sometimes ineffective or counterproductive.

For example, just because information is corrected does not mean that it no longer influences our beliefs and behaviour. Imagine reading a study that reports dangerous side effects from the MMR vaccine. Then you are told that the findings are totally unfounded and that it is an established fraud (which will remind you of the Wakefield case, see Chapter 4). You will still feel more suspicious of the vaccine than if you had never received information about the alleged side effects. This is known as the "lingering influence effect".[11] One explanation is that when the first (false) information was presented, our minds could not help but make a series of associations between this information and other knowledge or beliefs. For example, information about the adverse effects of the vaccine might be associated with beliefs about the pharmaceutical industry's disregard for patients or about the increasing frequency of autistic disorders in the population. In the presence of a correction, the subject will certainly question the false information targeted by the intervention, but will not integrate this correction with the other beliefs associated with the first information (for example, another reason should be found for the increase in autistic disorders).[12] For a correction to be effective, it is therefore important to do a real job of integrating the available information (original, false and corrected), which a simple rapid presentation of the correction fails to do.

In a similar vein, correcting false information often involves exposing people to the same problematic information. Yet the mere repetition of information, regardless of its degree of veracity, makes it subjectively more likely.[13] The fact that we have "heard it somewhere before" leads us to see it as more likely to be true. On the other hand, for a correction to be effective, it is also important that the correcting source is perceived as reliable. This is not necessarily the case! We know that a part of the population perceives the mainstream media with distrust and suspects (sometimes with reason) that they are driven by other concerns than the dissemination of proven information.

Based on this quick overview, the picture is rather mixed. Few solid studies (RCTs in particular) establish a clear and large-scale effect on the vaccination coverage of the samples studied. Effects on beliefs or intentions regarding vaccination are sometimes observed, but not necessarily translated into actual behaviour. While these approaches are interesting and sometimes promising, they are mostly focused on the individual. In reality, much more general and upstream interventions in the field of science, media and/or health education are undoubtedly necessary in order to build a real "psychological resilience" to (mis)information. How can we understand scientific information? How to identify reliable sources? How are the different actors producing discourses on the themes considered situated? What are their objectives, their networks? Unfortunately, there is little data on the effectiveness of this type of intervention, particularly in relation to vaccination.

ACTING ON INDIVIDUAL MOTIVATIONS

MOTIVATIONAL INTERVIEWING

As we saw in Chapter 2, self-motivation is a crucial ingredient in immunisation. One technique, motivational interviewing, aims precisely at influencing motivation. Developed to combat alcohol dependence, health professionals can also rely on the technique during individual meetings with people who experience vaccine hesitancy,[14] especially parents of children of vaccination age. Rather than seeking to "educate" parents in an asymmetrical relationship, the health professional will seek to motivate them to achieve certain health goals. It is based on developing an empathic relationship with the parents. For example, parents' fears and concerns about their child's vaccination will be identified without denouncing these fears as unfounded. Second, identify the target of change. In this case, it is, for example, a vaccine to be administered to the child. Thirdly, resistance to vaccination will be considered together, but the reasons for vaccinating children will also be explored. This is a prerequisite for the development of voluntary motivation. The parents will then see a real meaning in this vaccination and will fully identify with this decision.

Once the decision has been made, the next step is to identify ways to put it into practice. This technique has shown encouraging results for vaccination, particularly against HPV,[15] although there is still a lack of data establishing a robust effect of this technique on vaccination coverage. The only real obstacle is that the technique is resource-intensive, as it involves lengthy interviews with one or both parents and requires appropriate training of health staff.

EUROS FOR A SHOT

Another, radically different, technique is to influence not autonomous motivation but controlled motivation, by targeting the wallets of the reluctant. Indeed, during the COVID-19 pandemic, authorities in many countries, desperate for ideas to help overcome reluctance, offered various rewards to get people to come to vaccination centres. US President Joe Biden has offered $100 to anyone who agrees to be vaccinated. Several states (Maryland, Hong Kong) have offered raffles to win large sums of money. In Serbia and Sweden, cash was offered to those vaccinated.[16] These financial incentives were only introduced when the vaccination campaign was well underway, which can obviously create a sense of injustice among those who were vaccinated "for free". Moreover, this type of initiative can have perverse effects during a subsequent vaccination campaign if some decide to postpone vaccination in the hope of benefiting from a reward given to "latecomers".

One of the most successful studies on this topic is an RCT conducted in Sweden in May and July 2021 during the COVID-19 pandemic[17] and involving more than 8,000 unvaccinated people. People in the "incentive" group received SEK 200 (+/- EUR 20) if they were vaccinated within 30 days after the vaccine became available. In the control group, which did not receive this "reward", it was found that 71.6% of people were actually vaccinated at the end of this period. This percentage was 75.6% in the incentive group. A similar difference emerged with regard to participants' intentions, although the percentages were higher overall, namely 83.2 vs. 87.1%. In sum, relatively modest financial incentives could therefore be an effective solution, at least in the short term. However, other studies show less encouraging results. For example, before a COVID-19 vaccine was available, a German team[18] asked unvaccinated people to give their opinion on two possible choices: not to be vaccinated against COVID-19 (using a vaccine recommended for them) or to be vaccinated in exchange for a sum of money that could vary between 0 and 10,000 euros. In order to observe a significant increase in the rate of vaccination intentions, it was necessary to pay participants handsomely: a jackpot of 3,250 euros was indeed required! Even for 10,000 euros, almost 20% of the participants in this study did not want to be vaccinated (while more than 60% were willing without any incentive)!

This difference in results is probably due to the timing of the studies. Unlike the German study, the Swedish study was conducted when the vaccination campaign was well underway and the efficacy and safety of the proposed vaccines had been established. In addition, many people had already been vaccinated, creating a knock-on effect, which the financial incentive may have accentuated. This being said, the use of financial incentives is not without consequences on autonomous motivation, and thus on the long-term willingness to be vaccinated. We saw in Chapter 2 that autonomous motivation plays a key role in vaccination, unlike controlled motivation. According to the cognitive dissonance theory discussed in Chapter 3, it is likely that the existence of an incentive reduces autonomous motivation to vaccinate. This is especially relevant after the first dose of a vaccine. When vaccinated in the absence of a financial incentive, individuals will seek to match their attitude to their behaviour. People who were hesitant before vaccination are likely to 'rationalise' their choice to reduce dissonance. This is much less necessary when money or other rewards have been received in exchange for vaccination. However, this rationalisation promotes a real internalisation of the attitude towards vaccination, a condition for committing to a second or third dose. It is therefore not surprising that in one of our studies carried out as part of the Motivation Barometer,[19] the autonomous motivation felt with regard to the first dose of the COVID-19 vaccine remained predictive of the intention to accept the third dose several months later. However, the same influence was not found for controlled motivation.

MANDATORY VACCINATION AND OTHER INCENTIVES

Another method used to achieve sufficient vaccination coverage is obviously to make it compulsory, either for certain categories of the population (such as health care workers), or in a certain context (school, workplace, etc.), or for all "eligible" persons. This solution has not failed to arouse resistance, often based on legitimate legal arguments (such as the right to self-determination). Many people have protested against compulsory vaccination while at the same time declaring themselves personally in favour of vaccination (or even being vaccinated). It is therefore important to distinguish between vaccine hesitancy and opposition to compulsory vaccination!

What about it from a psychological point of view? Several psychological processes already mentioned are likely to come into play when such constraints are implemented. The first element to take into account concerns the implementation of the measure and, above all, the consequences foreseen for refusals. Indeed, compulsory vaccination means potential sanctions in the event of non-vaccination. However, the presence of such a sanction alone is often not enough to ensure that everyone is vaccinated. It is logistically and politically impossible in democratic societies to put in place a system of controls and penalties that is sufficiently effective and dissuasive to ensure that all those eligible for vaccination are vaccinated. Ultimately, compulsory vaccination is a psychological gamble: it will motivate people to get vaccinated.

Given this prerequisite, the presence of a sanction is tantamount to inducing a controlled motivation to be vaccinated. Such a motivation may well lead to action for fear of being sanctioned, but we have seen that this is not the most promising way of inducing adherence to vaccination, particularly in the long term. Mandatory vaccination can be seen as an admission of failure. The message is that if you can't be convinced, you are forced. More fundamentally, obligation and the associated sanctions are likely to be perceived as a threat to our freedom and to induce reactive behaviour, aimed at reaffirming our autonomy. This can lead to forms of anger and polarisation. In the context of a high-profile pandemic, and given that the discourse on vaccination is more than likely to be the subject of political mobilisation, this risk is very pronounced. Oppositions can more easily coalesce around a common discourse on mandatory vaccination.

In a study on attitudes towards vaccination carried out with a group of German students,[20] participants were asked to project themselves into a scenario in which a vaccine was available to deal with a potentially dangerous infectious disease and vaccination was presented as either compulsory or voluntary. Participants were then confronted with a second, very similar scenario, but in which vaccination was still voluntary. The study looked at the emotions felt when confronted with these scenarios and the decision made in the second situation. For participants with more negative attitudes towards vaccination, making vaccination compulsory at one point in time seemed to elicit more negative feelings (anger, reactance) that might jeopardise vaccination at a later time (when another dose would be needed, or another vaccine, etc.). In contrast, among those who were more favourable to vaccination at the start of the campaign, the initial obligation had little effect on subsequent vaccination. These results corroborate the role of reactance in response to the vaccination obligation, especially among those less willing to be vaccinated.

Another effect of obligation is to induce a prescriptive norm (see Chapter 3). When national authorities mandate vaccination, they signal to the citizens of that country that they must be vaccinated. This can therefore promote adherence indirectly by changing the perception of social norms.[21] Of course, all of this requires that decisions be made through a procedure and by authorities perceived as legitimate.[22]

In addition to compulsory vaccination, other forms of incentives exist. For example, access to certain places (restaurants, aeroplanes, cinemas, etc.) can be made conditional on vaccination or a test to prove that one is not infected. The effects of this type of measure are quite similar to those of compulsory vaccination in that it also affects controlled motivation. Unsurprisingly, such measures can create a sense of responsiveness and influence the perception of social norms. During the COVID-19 pandemic, data from the Motivation Barometer revealed that the perception of the "COVID-safe ticket", introduced in Belgium in the summer of 2021 (i.e. several months after the start of the vaccination campaign), was sharply contrasted between those who were vaccinated and those who were not. While the former group initially saw it as a way of ensuring greater health security by limiting the spread of the virus, the latter saw it as a threat to their autonomy as well as a way of making vaccination compulsory without admitting it outright. As the risk became less obvious, due to fewer severe cases and the predominance of variants perceived as less dangerous, the "COVID-safe ticket" was viewed more negatively and as "hypocritical" even by those vaccinated.[23] Also in a study conducted in January 2022 as part of the COVID-19 Pandemic Motivation Barometer,[24] the perception of risk also explained the attitude towards mandatory vaccination. Vaccinated people were more positive about compulsory vaccination than non-vaccinated people, but only if they perceived a high risk of infection.

ACTING ON SOCIAL PROCESSES

Following approaches focusing on beliefs and attitudes, we now turn to perspectives targeting social processes, including social norms, both descriptive and prescriptive, and altruistic motivations.

ACTING ON DESCRIPTIVE STANDARDS

As we saw in Chapter 3, one way to encourage immunisation is to act on social norms, both descriptive (what members of our community do) and prescriptive (what members of our community think we "should" do). Let us first consider descriptive norms. Individuals do not necessarily have a clear perception of the degree to which members of their group are complying with a particular social norm. In such situations, it is possible to vary the social norm. For example, telling hotel guests that "most guests keep the same towel from one night to the next for environmental reasons" is likely to encourage them to do the same.[25] A study of a large sample of Italian employees[26] tested this idea in the context of vaccination. These employees were informed of the rate of flu vaccination in their sub-region. This was actually modulated to appear high (e.g. 69%) or low (e.g. 13%). Subjects were then asked to estimate the likelihood that they would be vaccinated for the next winter. On average, this percentage was 5.5% higher in the high standard condition than in the low standard condition. Again, however, this study only looked at intentions and not at actual behaviour. To our knowledge, there are few RCTs examining the effect of descriptive social norms on vaccination behaviour. In contrast, a recent study[27] shows no effect of a message informing parents in Vermont of the state's consensus in favour of the vaccine on their willingness to vaccinate their own child.

ACTING ON PROSOCIAL MOTIVATIONS

In an epidemic, purely "selfish" motivations cannot be relied upon to achieve vaccine coverage. In the case of COVID-19, for example, the risk of serious infection resulting in hospitalisation was low for 18–30-year-olds. In the United States, hospitalisations were five times higher for those aged 65–74 and ten times higher for those aged 85 and older.[28] For elderly, therefore, vaccination helps to preserve their own health. This benefit can therefore be used as a "lever" to motivate these people to get vaccinated. However, to achieve sufficient vaccination coverage, and "herd immunity", younger people must also agree to be vaccinated. Among them, it is difficult to bet on purely selfish motivations. On the other hand, contributing to the health of more vulnerable people with whom one is likely to interact (a grandmother, an immunocompromised acquaintance, etc.) can be a strong incentive to get vaccinated. Research shows that this type of motivation is particularly likely to lead to vaccination if people are aware of the positive effect of vaccination on the community as a whole, and particularly on those at risk.[29] Such altruistic motivations are most likely to be present when individuals identify with the community in question and see it as an "ingroup".[30]

ACTING ON THE DOCTOR'S RECOMMENDATION

We have seen that health care professionals enjoy a high level of trust. Their word can thus be the source of a prescriptive norm. In a study conducted by a Czech team,[31] it was found that a large part of the population has a truncated perception of what the medical community thinks about vaccination: doctors are seen as more divided than they actually are. Indeed, "anti-vaccination" discourses often appeal to figures from the medical world. While a survey of more than 9,000 doctors showed a very high level of consensus on the value of vaccination against COVID-19 (more than 90% were in favour), this level was estimated at an average of 60% by ordinary Czechs. The study then included an intervention on a large group of Czechs. One half of the group, the experimental group, was informed about the existence of a consensus in the medical community about vaccination by showing them (among other things) charts from the preliminary study. A control group was not given any information on this subject. An effect of this intervention was observed in the medium term. Four months later, the experimental group was more likely to have been vaccinated than the control group (the difference was around 5%). This shows the power of prescriptive norms (doctors recommend vaccination) combined with descriptive norms within the medical community (agreement on vaccination).

A smaller German study provides a very interesting insight into the role of the family doctor in the vaccination decision.[32] The participants recruited in April 2021, were first asked to indicate what type of recommendations their doctor had already made to them concerning vaccination. They were then asked to imagine that their family doctor invited them to be vaccinated against COVID-19. In addition, half of the participants were asked to imagine that their doctor had been vaccinated against COVID-19 and the other half that this was not the case. As expected, imagining that the doctor had been vaccinated influenced vaccination intentions. Presumably, the doctor's behaviour is seen as indicative of a social norm to which subjects conform. There was also much more reluctance when the doctor recommended not to be vaccinated than the other way around. Participants who received no recommendation fell between these two extremes. These results confirm that the doctor's recommendation can have a very important effect on the willingness to be vaccinated. However, it cannot be ruled out that the relationship between doctor's recommendation and intention to vaccinate is partly due to a selection effect (i.e. people who are unfavourable to vaccination are more likely to opt for a doctor who is not a vaccine supporter).

How should doctors proceed to ensure that their views are heard? An American study explored this question with parents of infants in preparation for their children's vaccination.[33] Interviews between 111 parents of children under 20 months of age and a paediatrician were filmed and recorded during a routine visit. Half of these parents had been identified on the basis of a questionnaire as being hesitant about vaccination. It was found that the way in which the paediatricians communicated had a very important effect on the parents' reaction. The scientific team then looked in particular at what they termed "resistance", i.e. reacting negatively to the doctor's recommendation to vaccinate their child. Resistance to vaccination was much higher (74%) when the recommendation was made in an assertive manner ("We need to do some vaccinations") than when the paediatrician adopted a participatory style ("Do you want to do some vaccinations today?"): 17%. And when parents "resisted", the doctor's insistence was enough to "convert" 50% of these resistant parents. In other words, even when they are hesitant, parents tend to comply with the doctor's authority. Hesitation does not necessarily correspond to a firmly held feeling, but sometimes reflects a simple lack of knowledge, an uncertainty that can be swept away by a trustworthy authority. Here again, the doctor's discourse appears as a "prescriptive norm" to which parents conform. Once again, caution should be exercised with regard to the conclusions of this study as it is not an RCT.

ACTING DIRECTLY ON BEHAVIOUR

The interventions considered so far are aimed at changing people's perceptions of vaccination. Some approaches are more individual and others focus on more collective processes. What about interventions that aim to encourage reluctant people to move from intention to action? Rather than modulating the underlying attitudes of individuals, the aim is to facilitate "action". In line with the 3Cs model discussed in Chapter 2, they aim to address "complacency" and "comfort" rather than "confidence".

Overall, these approaches are part of the *nudging* framework.[34] "Nudge" refers to a set of methods aimed at influencing behaviour without limiting choice or providing incentives. One example is to put a picture of a fly on the opening of a urinal, a technique that encourages people to be as precise as possible, thus increasing hygiene and reducing the workload of cleaning staff. Another example is to make fruit more readily available than chocolate bars in shop displays to encourage healthy eating.

The first type of intervention is simply to remind people who are eligible for vaccination that they are eligible through various information channels. This could be a card sent by post or dropped in the mailbox, an e-mail, an SMS, etc. In the same spirit, one could send a card to a person who is not eligible for vaccination. In the same vein, a message could be sent to those who did not get vaccinated at the scheduled time. In a study conducted in California during the COVID-19 pandemic,[35] the local health agency reminded people that they could get vaccinated and provided a link to easily register for an appointment. This increased vaccination by about 5% compared to a control group. Remarkably, a variation of this message that emphasised that the vaccine was "right for you" was even more effective. As we saw in Chapter 4, many people are reluctant to be vaccinated not because they are fundamentally opposed to vaccination, but because they believe they have unique characteristics that may cause specific side effects in themselves (or their child). Even when formatted to this extent, this type of message therefore promotes vaccination.

Such messages will be all the more effective if vaccination is presented as the "default" option ("it's time for your flu shot" rather than "do you want to be vaccinated against flu?"[36]). In this way, vaccination appears as a social norm (and therefore all the more legitimate, especially for people who would not have crystallised attitudes on this issue). On the other hand, it requires a greater effort to give it up. It is always easier to go with the flow than to go against it! For example, if vaccination of school-age children is scheduled during a medical visit unless the parents (duly informed) object, vaccination coverage is likely to be much higher than if it is scheduled only at the parents' request.

In the same vein, offering registration systems in which people specify a time and date to be vaccinated greatly increases the likelihood of actually getting the vaccine.[37] This is why appointment-based reminder systems are so effective. Interventions that target knowledge about immunisation are often not successful because they do not provide a concrete opportunity to be immunised at a specific time and place. It therefore seems crucial that information approaches are complemented by nudges.

BALANCE SHEET

What can be learned from this overview of the different interventions that can influence vaccination decisions? A recent review of the literature on this topic[38] suggests that the interventions with the clearest empirical support are

- act via doctor's recommendation;
- encourage action (in particular by means of "nudges");
- provide incentives for people to get vaccinated;
- impose obligation (educational or professional).

On the other hand, Brewer argues that there is less clear evidence to support the role of interventions based on participants' beliefs, individual motivations or attitudes, or even on descriptive norms. This does not necessarily mean that these approaches are without merit. Consider the case of descriptive norms. As we saw in Chapter 3, the effect of social norms on a wide range of behaviours has been repeatedly and overwhelmingly established, and some studies that are correlational, or rely on measures of intention rather than behaviour, suggest effects on vaccination. However, the literature remains too sparse in experimental studies (RCTs) to support the effectiveness of this approach on vaccination. Such research is needed before strong conclusions can be drawn about the (in)effectiveness of this approach.

Again, it should be remembered that each study is set in a particular cultural and historical context and concerns specific vaccines and interventions. They are therefore not always easily comparable. This means that good quality studies that compare different interventions are particularly valuable. For example, the Swedish study on financial incentives[193] is particularly interesting because it contrasts with others that deserve a few lines. One study looked at altruistic motivations (by asking participants to name four people in their lives who would benefit from vaccination). Two others focused on beliefs and attitudes. In one, participants were asked to take part in a quiz about the vaccine (this provided information about its effectiveness). In the other, they were asked to name arguments that would convince another person to get vaccinated. This was also aimed at attitude-behaviour consistency (see Chapter 3) with the hope that, to minimise cognitive dissonance, participants who had expressed such arguments would then want to be vaccinated. All three interventions were found to have no effect on vaccination intentions or on vaccination itself (within 30 days), while financial incentives were found to be the most effective, with a 4% increase. Again, these results show a limited effect of the interventions on beliefs/attitudes and social motivations.

A vaccination campaign needs to combine different approaches. In the light of the above, the first priority from a psychological point of view seems to be to facilitate vaccination for those who are already independently motivated (and who will often also be the most at risk). Nudging can be particularly valuable in this regard. It can be updated with (among other things) reminders, but also with initiatives to make vaccination closer, easier and cheaper. For example, there have been 'vaccine buses' that have travelled through certain neighbourhoods – saving people the trouble of having to go to a vaccination centre. Similarly, registering for vaccinations should be easy (either through a well-designed website or a phone call if it is not possible to go to the centre without an appointment). The success of such an approach can then create a "ripple effect".

We have seen that general messages about the safety of vaccines and the risks posed by the disease are not very effective. The content of the message is often less important than the source of the message. For a communication to work, the communicator must generate trust. In this respect, and at the risk of repeating ourselves, the role of the family doctor and, more generally, of the health care professionals who are in direct contact with hesitant people (pharmacists, nurses, etc.) is absolutely crucial. It is therefore important to give them the tools to dialogue with people who hesitate. Training these staff, especially in motivational interviewing, can be very valuable. When other sources of communication are used (scientific experts, political authorities, etc.), they must be seen to be representative of the audiences they address, whether in terms of gender, age or ethnocultural background. Indeed, as we have seen, trust is also nurtured by the feeling that the person speaking belongs to the same community as oneself (see Chapter 3).

It should be remembered that while financial incentives can be used with some success to "boost" vaccination among reluctant groups, they are not without perverse effects (feeling of injustice, reduced autonomous motivation). In the long term, it remains very important to rely on the altruistic motivations of individuals. This requires an awareness of the fact that vaccination is part of a "social contract" that allows the whole of society to function on a basis that benefits everyone. The leitmotif here is undoubtedly to ensure that the population understands that the collective and the individual work hand in hand. As with the Highway Code, which is restrictive in many respects but also offers the possibility of travelling with maximum safety, vaccination is a behaviour that requires people to agree to play the game so that the collective benefit can be achieved at the lowest cost. In this regard, the public needs to be informed of the many altruistic and cooperative behaviours that emerge in a pandemic situation. Journalists would do well to focus on exemplary behaviour, which is in fact in the vast majority, and not just on "raids on pasta or toilet paper" or clandestine gatherings during periods of containment. The media, which has often been accused of "anxiety-provoking" communication, has a decisive role to play in supporting the population in the efforts it makes.

NOTES

1 Böhm, R., Betsch, C., Litovsky, Y., Sprengholz, P., Brewer, N. T., Chapman, G., Leask, J., Loewenstein, G., Scherzer, M., Sunstein, C. R., & Kirchler, M. (2022). Crowdsourcing interventions to promote uptake of COVID-19 booster vaccines. *EClinicalMedicine*, 53.

2 Funder, D. C., & Ozer, D. J. (2019). Evaluating effect size in psychological research: Sense and nonsense. *Advances in Methods and Practices in Psychological Science*, 2(2), 156–168.

3 Nasiru, S.-G., Aliyu, G. G., Gasasira, A., Aliyu, M. H., Zubair, M., Mandawari, S. U., Waziri, H., Nasidi, A., & El-Kamary, S. S. (2012). Breaking community barriers to polio vaccination in northern Nigeria: The impact of a grass roots mobilization campaign (Majigi). *Pathogens and Global Health*, 106(3), 166–171.

4 Eitze, S., Heinemeier, D., Schmid-Küpke, N. K., & Betsch, C. (2021). Decreasing vaccine hesitancy with extended health knowledge: Evidence from a longitudinal randomized controlled trial. *Health Psychology*, 40(2), 77–88. https://doi.org/10.1037/hea0001045.

5 Brewer, N. T., Chapman, G. B., Rothman, A. J., Leask, J., & Kempe, A. (2017). Increasing vaccination: Putting psychological science into action. *Psychological Science in the Public Interest*, 18(3), 149–207.

6 Betsch, C., & Böhm, R. (2016). Detrimental effects of introducing partial compulsory vaccination: Experimental evidence. *The European Journal of Public Health*, 26(3), 378–381.

7 Morbée, S., Waterschoot, J., Yzerbyt, V., Klein, O., Luminet, O., Schmitz, M., Van den Bergh, O., Van Oost, P., De Craene, S., & Vansteenkiste, M. (2022).

Personal and contextual determinants of COVID-19 vaccination intention: A vignette study. *Expert Review of Vaccines*, 21(10), 1475–1485.

8 Compton, J., van der Linden, S., Cook, J., & Basol, M. (2021). Inoculation theory in the post-truth era: Extant findings and new frontiers for contested science, misinformation, and conspiracy theories. *Social and Personality Psychology Compass*, 15(6).

9 Vivion, M., Anassour Laouan Sidi, E., Betsch, C., Dionne, M., Dubé, E., Driedger, S. M., Gagnon, D., Graham, J., Greyson, D., Hamel, D., Lewandowsky, S., MacDonald, N., Malo, B., Meyer, S. B., Schmid, P., Steenbeek, A., van der Linden, S., Verger, P., Witteman, H. O., & Yesilada, M. (2022). Prebunking messaging to inoculate against COVID-19 vaccine misinformation: An effective strategy for public health. *Journal of Communication in Healthcare*, 15(3), 232–242.

10 Carey, J. M., Guess, A. M., Loewen, P. J., Merkley, E., Nyhan, B., Phillips, J. B., & Reifler, J. (2022). The ephemeral effects of fact-checks on COVID-19 misperceptions in the United States, Great Britain and Canada. *Nature Human Behaviour*, 6(2).

11 Johnson, H. M., & Seifert, C. M. (1994). Sources of the continued influence effect: When misinformation in memory affects later inferences. *Journal of Experimental Psychology: Learning, Memory, and Cognition*, 20(6), 1420–1436.

12 Ecker, U. K. H., Lewandowsky, S., Cook, J., Schmid, P., Fazio, L. K., Brashier, N., Kendeou, P., Vraga, E. K., & Amazeen, M. A. (2022). The psychological drivers of misinformation belief and its resistance to correction. *Nature Reviews Psychology*, 1(1), 13–29.

13 Hasher, L., Goldstein, D., & Toppino, T. (1977). Frequency and the conference of referential validity. *Journal of Verbal Learning and Verbal Behavior*, 16(1), 107–112.

14 Gagneur, A. (2020). Motivational interviewing: A powerful tool to address vaccine hesitancy. *Canada Communicable Disease Report*, 46(4), 93–97.

15 Dempsey, A.F.; Pyrznawoski, J.; Lockhart, S.; Barnard, J.; Campagna, E.J.; Garrett, K.; Fisher, A.; Dickinson, L.M.; O'Leary, S.T. (2018). Effect of a health care professional communication training intervention on adolescent human papillomavirus vaccination: A cluster randomized clinical trial. *JAMA Pediatrics*, 172(5), e180016.

16 Klingert, L. (2021). 'Jabs for kebabs': The art of coronavirus vaccine persuasion. *POLITICO*. www.politico.eu/article/coronavirus-vaccine-reward-europe-skepticism.

17 Campos-Mercade, P., Meier, A. N., Schneider, F. H., Meier, S., Pope, D., & Wengström, E. (2021). Monetary incentives increase COVID-19 vaccinations. *Science*, 374(6569), 879–882.

18 Sprengholz, P., Eitze, S., Felgendreff, L., Korn, L., & Betsch, C. (2021). Money is not everything: Experimental evidence that payments do not increase willingness to be vaccinated against COVID-19. *Journal of Medical Ethics*, 47(8), 547–548.

19 Waterschoot, J., Van Oost, P., Schmitz, M., Morbée, S., Klein, O., Vansteenkiste, M., Luminet, O., Van den Bergh, O., & Yzerbyt, V. (2022). *The role of vaccination motivation in people's intention to accept a booster dose*. Unpublished manuscript.

20 Sprengholz, P., Felgendreff, L., Böhm, R., & Betsch, C. (2022). Vaccination policy reactance: Predictors, consequences, and countermeasures. *Journal of Health Psychology*, 27(6), 1394–1407.

21 Zeev-Wolf, M., & Mentovich, A. (2022). The influence of the legislative and judicial branches on moral judgment and norm perception with the special case of judicial intervention. *Regulation & Governance*, 16(4), 1211–1232.

22 Tyler, T. R. (1989). The psychology of procedural justice: A test of the group-value model. *Journal of Personality and Social Psychology*, 57(5), 830–838.

23 Goubert, L., Klein, O., Luminet, O., Morbée, S., Schmitz, M., Van den Bergh, O., Van Oost, P., Vansteenkiste, M., Yzerbyt, V., & Waterschoot, J. (2022). *Motivation, well-being and attitudes towards vaccination in the time of the omicron. Motivation Barometer Report, 39*. Belgium: Ghent University. https://motivationbarometer.com/en/portfolio-item/rapport-39-motivatie-welbevinden-en-vaccinatie-attitudes-in-omikron-tijden/.

24 Brisbois, M., Schmitz, M., Vansteenkiste, M., Yzerbyt, V., Van Oost, P., Morbée, S., Waterschoot, J., Luminet, O., Van den Bergh, O., Raemdonck, E., & Klein, O. (2023). *Attitudes towards mandatory vaccination and the COVID certificate as a function of vaccination status and risk perception: A vignette-based study*. Unpublished manuscript. Belgium: Université libre de Bruxelles.

25 Goldstein, N. J., Cialdini, R. B., & Griskevicius, V. (2008). A room with a viewpoint: Using social norms to motivate environmental conservation in hotels. *Journal of Consumer Research*, 35(3), 472–482.

26 Belle, N., & Cantarelli, P. (2021). Nudging public employees through descriptive social norms in healthcare organizations. *Public Administration Review*, 81(4), 589–598.

27 Clayton, K., Finley, C., Flynn, D. J., Graves, M., & Nyhan, B. (2021). Evaluating the effects of vaccine messaging on immunization intentions and behavior: Evidence from two randomized controlled trials in Vermont. *Vaccine*, 39(40), 5909–5917.

28 Center for Disease Control and Prevention. (2022). *Risk for COVID-19 infection, hospitalization, and death by age group*. www.cdc.gov/coronavirus/2019-ncov/covid-data/investigations-discovery/hospitalization-death-by-age.html.

29 Betsch, C., Böhm, R., Korn, L., & Holtmann, C. (2017). On the benefits of explaining herd immunity in vaccine advocacy. *Nature Human Behaviour*, 1, 56.

30 Levine, M., Prosser, A., Evans, D., & Reicher, S. (2005). Identity and emergency intervention: How social group membership and inclusiveness of group boundaries shape helping behavior. *Personality & Social Psychology Bulletin*, 31(4), 443–453.

31 Bartoš, V., Bauer, M., Cahlíková, J., & Chytilová, J. (2022). Communicating doctors' consensus persistently increases COVID-19 vaccinations. *Nature*, 606(7914), 542–549.

32 Sprengholz, P., Korn, L., Eitze, S., Siegers, R., & Betsch, C. (2022). *What the doctor ordered: Family doctors' recommendations strongly impact patients' COVID-19 vaccination intentions*. Unpublished manuscript.

33 Opel, D. J., Heritage, J., Taylor, J. A., Mangione-Smith, R., Salas, H. S., DeVere, V., Zhou, C., & Robinson, J. D. (2013). The architecture of provider-parent vaccine discussions at health supervision visits. *Pediatrics*, 132(6), 1037–1046.

34 Sunstein, C. R., & Thaler, R. H. (2010). *Nudges. Emotions, habits, behaviours: How to inspire the right decisions*. Paris: Vuibert.

35 Dai, H., Saccardo, S., Han, M. A., Roh, L., Raja, N., Vangala, S., Modi, H., Pandya, S., Sloyan, M., & Croymans, D. M. (2021). Behavioural nudges increase COVID-19 vaccinations. *Nature*, 597, art. 7876.

36 Brewer, N. T. *et al.* (2017). *Op. cit.* p. 177.

37 Milkman, K. L., Beshears, J., Choi, J. J., Laibson, D., & Madrian, B. C. (2011). Using implementation intentions prompts to enhance influenza vaccination rates. *Proceedings of the National Academy of Sciences*, 108(26), 10415–10420.

38 Brewer, N. T. (2021). What works to increase vaccination uptake. *Academic Pediatrics*, 21(4S), S9–S16.

CONCLUSION

It is tempting to see vaccine hesitancy as a societal disease that should be eradicated, much like smallpox. As we have seen in the preceding pages, this view obscures the fact that vaccine hesitancy is not just an individual or social dysfunction. It is itself rooted in social representations, often specific to communities, periods and vaccines. Given the polymorphic nature of vaccine hesitancy, there is no universal "medicine" for this phenomenon. Furthermore, using the metaphor of disease, it is assumed that vaccine hesitancy is necessarily "unhealthy". However, it may reflect legitimate questions about the relevance of certain vaccines or the way the vaccination campaign is conducted.

Seeing vaccine hesitancy as a disease, or the consequence of an "infodemic", illustrates our tendency to approach psychosocial phenomena from a medical perspective. In March 2020, when the first health measures against the COVID-19 pandemic were introduced by the Belgian authorities, we were concerned about a purely medical approach focusing on the transmission of the virus. This tended to obscure the social relations in which this transmission took place. In particular, the term "social distancing" made us bristle at a time when, more than ever, and as many research studies in the human

DOI: 10.4324/9781032665429-7

sciences suggested, we needed social proximity. It would have been so much simpler to talk about physical distancing. "Far from the eyes, close to the heart", we entitled our column. More than two years later, it seems to us that the importance of social relations, and of the various sciences that study them, in the apprehension and management of diseases is more widely recognised by the authorities and by public opinion.

First, we reviewed a range of psychological determinants of vaccination with behavioural intention as the most direct antecedent. This is directly conditioned by motivation. A large body of research supports the crucial role of one form of motivation, autonomous motivation, in the emergence of this intention. Indeed, vaccination must be experienced as a decision that is freely consented to and assumed. Conversely, when it is perceived as undermining a feeling of autonomy (through restrictive measures), we observe reactance and a refusal to consent. We then looked at factors further upstream in the behaviour, and in particular at trust. Confidence in the safety and efficacy of the vaccine is of course a crucial determinant of motivation and helps shape positive attitudes towards vaccination. We have seen how this confidence can be undermined by fake news about the risks of vaccination to human health or by conspiracy theories that are more general. Such fake news are widely disseminated and, via the "truth bias", are likely to influence beliefs about vaccination, trust in it and vaccination intentions. This is also done through emotions such as anger.

However, the decision to be vaccinated is also based on trust in a multiplicity of actors. In this respect, the role of health care professionals who are in direct contact with hesitant people (family doctors, pharmacists, nurses, etc.) should be emphasised. All of these stakeholders need to have tools that allow them to dialogue with people who are hesitant. The work examined in the preceding pages highlights the importance of being able to train these staff in motivational interviewing. As for the other sources of communication (scientific experts, political authorities, etc.), it is important that the audiences to whom they are addressed see them as representative, whether in terms of gender, age or ethno-cultural background. There is nothing more valuable for building trust than to see that the source of a message is part of the same community as oneself.

Indeed, behind the individual who chooses or not to be vaccinated lies a multitude of social affiliations and ties that help shape his or her decision. It is through this prism that we have considered the vaccination decision. In particular, we have articulated the radical thesis of social identity theory that individuals' identities evolve according to the social context and communities that best allow them to be understood *hic et nunc*. These affiliations guide behaviour through the influence of social norms and shared representations within the community. This is what we have seen through the knock-on effect. They can also encourage mistrust and conflict by making a behaviour (to be vaccinated or not) an identity marker. Vaccination is also a form of social contract – in which everyone makes an effort for the community and expects to be treated well in return, whatever other affiliations they may have. Of course, this does not prevent some people from "going it alone", taking advantage of the efforts of others without actually doing anything themselves.

What must be at the heart of the approach is that the population should be able to take full measure of the fact that the collective and the individual are linked and that it is undesirable to function as a particular being whose health is unlikely to be permanently altered by illness. As has been said, the reason why the Highway Code is so valuable for the movement of people on public highways, whether they are motorists, cyclists or mere pedestrians, is that it is based on a set of constraints. In the same way, vaccination requires compliance with certain recommendations in order to reap the collective benefit that is hoped for. In this context, there is nothing like highlighting the healthy behaviours, which are the most popular. Of course, we can understand the temptation in the press to focus citizens' attention on the massive and absurd purchases of toilet paper or to highlight the more or less thunderous deviations from the authorities' recommendations on health measures. However, altruism and cooperation prevail in times of pandemic, and the media can undoubtedly contribute to appeasement rather than cultivate anxiety and fear. If we are to maintain long-term motivation for vaccination in our democratic societies (the problem is different in authoritarian societies where outright coercion is the common solution), identification with this larger community – supra-ordinate, as the social identity approach calls it – is essential. It is therefore a difficult task to consider the many reasons for seeing our singular situation, or that of the minority to which we (belong), as fundamentally different from that of the rest of the population. All in all, an immunisation campaign is an experiment in managing diversity and even more so in managing inclusion on a large scale.

Between the decisions to be vaccinated or not, there is a wide range of postures ("maybe", "not right away", "not with that vaccine", etc.). Moreover, the same response can correspond to very different psychological realities. Finally, and above all, it is important not to consider these positions as fixed. Depending on events (changes in epidemiological indicators, the roll-out of a vaccination campaign, for example), attitudes and motivations are likely to change. In Belgium, it has been observed that most people who, before the vaccination campaign, were adamant about not wanting to be vaccinated eventually decided to do so. More generally, it would be not only insulting but also misleading to consider that people who are against vaccination are more stupid, irrational or even delusional than others. The latter are also influenced by the psychosocial processes we have described (attitudes, motivation, conformism, social identities, social representations, rumours, etc.). In view of these elements, stigmatising people who hesitate as a "plague" on society is probably the best way to further entrench them in a posture of distrust towards authorities who (from their point of view) do not respect them.

It is clear that taking human behaviour into account, whether in its individual, interpersonal, intergroup or ideological dimensions, seems to us to be essential in order to optimise the responses to be given to major challenges such as the COVID-19 pandemic, but also to others that will arise in the coming years. Indeed, how can we imagine that we can apprehend the upheavals linked to the global warming that is taking shape before our eyes or to the collapse of biodiversity without integrating the populations into the equation? It is an illusion to believe that we can prevent, accompany and remedy the inevitable damage of what is now called the Anthropocene, the period during which humans rule the earth at the risk of compromising their own survival, solely through medical or technological responses. Through this book, we hope to have made a small contribution to raising awareness of the indispensable nature of the human and social sciences and, in particular, the psychological sciences in the search for solutions.

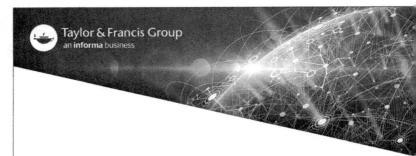

Printed in the United States
by Baker & Taylor Publisher Services